BRAIN WORKOUT

Also by Arthur Winter and Ruth Winter:

Eat Right, Be Bright

BRAIN WORKOUT

Easy Ways to Power UP Your Memory,
Sensory Perception, and Intelligence

Arthur Winter, MD
and
Ruth Winter, MS

ASJA Press
New York   Lincoln   Shanghai

Brain Workout
Easy Ways to Power Up Your Memory, Sensory Perception, and Intelligence

ASJA Press
an imprint of iUniverse, Inc.

For information address:
iUniverse, Inc.
2021 Pine Lake Road, Suite 100
Lincoln, NE 68512
www.iuniverse.com

Originally published by St. Martin's Press

A previous edition of this work was published under the title *Build Your Brain Power* by St. Martin's Press, 1986.

ISBN: 0-595-30092-8

Printed in the United States of America

To Robin, Craig, Grant, Jonathan,
Samantha, Hunter, Katelynd

Contents

Foreword   ix

1. You Can Gain Brain Power   1
2. Sense and Sensitivity: How to Perfect Your Sensory
   Perception   11
3. Enhancing Coordination and Motor Skills   46
4. Brain Aerobics: Physical Exercises That Go to Your Head   61
5. Fine-Tuning Your Brain with Music   71
6. How to Improve Your Memory   90
7. Expand Your Capacity to Learn   109
8. Free Your Creativity   122
9. Food and Supplements to Fuel Your Brain   135
10. Protecting Your Brain Against Potentially Harmful
    Chemicals   161
11. Chemicals for the Mind: The Search for Memory
    Enhancers   171
12. Stop Stress from Short-Circuiting Your Brain   180
13. Do You Need Professional Help?   204
14. Prepare for Your Future   209

Notes   213
Glossary   231
Index   241

Foreword

I am a "brain mechanic," a neurosurgeon who for years repaired damaged brains. Many of my patients were awake during the operations, because the brain itself feels no pain. Some of these people could actually converse and reminisce while I repaired a blood vessel or removed a tumor from their brains.

The organ has never ceased to amaze me. Some patients with severe damage that caused them to be paralyzed and unable to speak made excellent recoveries by unshakeable willpower and a willingness to pursue rehabilitation. Many with far less damage remained lethargic and did not participate in their rehabilitation or their intellectual growth. This made it quite evident to me that there is far more to brain power than anatomy. Motivation and enthusiasm can overcome seemingly insurmountable barriers.

New research is proving that much of the deterioration in memory and intellectual function we at one time blamed on age is actually due to disuse. If you don't take action, your brain, like your muscles, may become "flabby."

When we first wrote *Build Your Brain Power* in the mid-1980s, it was a rather novel idea that you could prevent or delay the degeneration of intellect even into very old age with mental and physical exercises and an understanding of the effects of behavior on your most important organ. Since then, much scientific evidence has been gathered to support this theory.

One of the most fruitful areas of the recent research, and the one upon which we have based this book, concerns brain potential. It is now clear that your brain can be developed and maintained to a degree, at any age. The "degree" often depends on the one thing that no one yet understands clearly—motivation.

There is an observation about which there is unanimous agreement among neurological researchers—humans use only a fraction of their brain's true potential!

In *Brain Workout* we describe the latest research and techniques available to power up your memory, sensory perception, and intelligence. We hope to stimulate you and to help you develop and maintain your brain to near its maximum capacities.

We can present the facts, theories, and techniques, but it is up to you to make the effort.

Arthur Winter, M.D., and Ruth Winter, M.S.
New Jersey Neurological Institute
Livingston, New Jersey

BRAIN
WORKOUT

1

You Can Gain Brain Power

"Education consists of modification in the central nervous system. For this experience, the cell elements are peculiarly fitted. They are plastic in the sense that their connections are not rigidly fixed, and they re-member . . . By virtue of these powers, the cells can adjust themselves to new surroundings."[1]

The above was written in 1895 by Henry Donaldson, professor of neurology at the University of Chicago. What Professor Donaldson surmised at the time is being proven today over and over again by high-tech diagnostic instruments: You can increase your brain power!

Steven E. Petersen, Ph.D., an associate professor of neurology at Washington University School of Medicine, St. Louis, Missouri, and Randy L. Buckner, a doctoral student, are studying the brain using a PET scanner (positron emission tomography). The PET scan was one of the first methods that allowed scientists to study the working brain in live humans at various times and under different circumstances. Unlike CAT scans (computerized axial tomography, or computerized X-rays), which show the shape and anatomy of the brain, PET scans reveal the biochemical changes taking place as the living brain goes about its continuous business of interacting with the world around it.

The Washington University researchers say, "Just as our muscles require more blood when they do work, so does the brain. If we wanted to know which muscles are used to lift a weight, we might have some-one lift the weight and see which muscles get bigger. To figure out which areas of the brain are used for language, we have subjects do a language test and see which areas of the brain increase their blood flow."[2]

The Washington University PET scanner can localize active areas as tiny as three millimeters—about the size of a dot on dice. The scanner can even detect differences between how men and women think.[3] Marcus E. Raichle, M.D., professor of neurology and radiology,

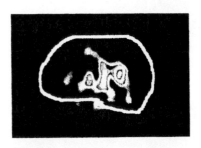

Frame 1: Hearing

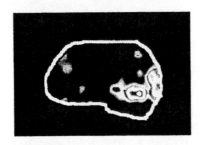

Frame 3: Seeing

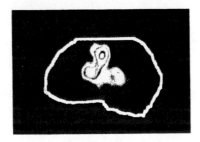

Frame 2: Speaking

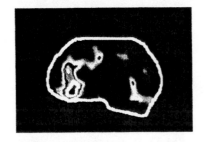

Frame 4: Thinking

PET SCAN
Positron Emission
Tomography (PET)
Imaging modality demonstrates quantitative information about biochemical and physiologic processes such as thinking, vision, hearing, memory, music, language.

and his group, also at Washington University, found by using PET scans why practicing causes a piano piece or a tennis stroke to become "automatic." When learning a task, Dr. Raichle and his colleagues observed, a person uses a "novel" circuit specifically designed for handling new tasks. After practice, though, there is a switch to a second circuit in a different location in the brain that handles learned tasks. As a task is repeated, it becomes *automatic;* that is, requiring less attention and little activity in the area of the brain previously involved. Other areas of the brain become more active in the automatic state. In the study, the switch took less than fifteen minutes of practice.

The Washington University investigators believe that their study shows how the brain might free itself from having to fret over mundane tasks—like shifting a car gear at the right time or walking—in order to devote energy to other endeavors. This might be the brain's way of conserving attention—a precious resource.

Can the PET scan show the difference between how a young brain and an old one thinks?

Ranjan Duara, M.D., working with his former colleagues at the National Institutes of Health (NIH), used a PET scan to study the difference between the metabolism of younger and older brains. Metabolism refers to the brain's use of its fuel, most commonly sugars, to operate. During the sessions volunteers between the ages of twenty and eighty were injected with two radioactive substances. Their ears were plugged and their eyes masked, but they were instructed not to fall asleep, just to relax. Forty-five minutes later, they placed their heads in holders that fit inside metal cylinders.

The volunteers were given a series of geometric designs to copy at their leisure and a few other noncompetitive tasks. As they performed their assignments while the PET "watched," doctors monitored where in the brain the radioactive-tagged glucose was being consumed, thus pinpointing the area of the brain being used to "perform" or to "think" about the task.[4]

"There was no significant difference in metabolism between the healthy older brains and the healthy younger ones in a resting state," Duara said. "There were some variations noted more commonly in older subjects, but they were not universal. Some men in their eighties had exactly the same brain metabolism as much younger men, while some younger men showed the changes usually observed in older brains."[5]

A tremendous revolution has taken place in how science thinks about the brain. New information gathered by a wide variety of experts, including neuroscientists who have been able to listen to a single brain cell "talking," have found that there is very little difference in functional capacity between the brains of healthy young people and healthy older people.

There are common age changes in the brain, of course, just as there are wrinkles on the skin. The MRI scan does show that there is a degree of atrophy, and the brains of most seventy-year-olds are lighter in weight than those of the average twenty-year-old. The joints and muscles of a forty-five-year-old are not, on the average, as flexible as those of a twenty-five-year-old, either. However, just as a trained and motivated thirty-seven-year-old Carlos Lopes of Portugal could beat men in their early twenties in an Olympic marathon, older people of the same basic intelligence as twenty-year-olds outperform them because the seniors have continued to train their brains, and have acquired more experience.

As with wrinkles and other physical changes that occur with age, age changes in the brain don't happen to everyone at the same time or to the same degree.

This point was made clear when Congress asked the National Institutes of Health and the Secretary of Transportation in 1979 to study the "Age 60 rule," which forced commercial pilots to retire. After ten months, the study committee concluded that "variability [in the effects of aging] within an age group is often nearly as great as variability among age groups, and that usually no single age emerges as a point of sharp decline . . . Available evidence suggests that on the average at least some of the skills necessary to the highest level of safety deteriorate with age. However, there is great variation among individuals within any age group."[6]

The long-accepted belief that we all lose a great many brain cells as we age was based on faulty research. Marian Diamond, Ph.D., professor of anatomy at the University of California at Irvine, explained why: "They took the brain of a healthy eight-year-old and compared it to the brain of a sick eighty-year-old and found there was a 10 to 20 percent decrease in the surface area and that was interpolated that we all lose one hundred thousand brain cells after the age of thirty. People accepted this. But the brains they studied were inactive, degenerate brains, and naturally you are going to see a loss of cells. If you look at healthy [older] brains, you don't find this loss."[7]

The brain, by weight alone, is 90 percent of the central nervous system. There is also a long extension of the brain descending inside the backbone, known as the spinal cord. From both the brain and the spinal cord, nerves go out to the sensory organs, such as the eyes, ears, and nose. Nerves also go out to muscles, skin, and all the other organs of the body.

One of the major functions of the central nervous system is communication within its various parts and with the outside world. The signals that converse within the brain are electrical and chemical in nature. Within individual nerve cells or neurons, the conversations are predominantly *electrical.* The signals that are transmitted from one nerve to another, conversely, are largely *chemical.*

As new discoveries about the human brain are made within a wide variety of disciplines, old beliefs and research conclusions are being proved wrong. Until quite recently, for example, communication between the nerves was thought to occur only at specialized junctions between cells called *synapses.* It has now been discovered that nerves not only produce chemicals that affect adjoining nerves but can issue substances that travel throughout the body, affecting other nerves at distant sites. It was also believed that only one chemical was active at one synapse. Now it has been observed that several chemicals may be sent out and received at a single site. Furthermore, it was assumed that the axon, the long "wire" that carries the nerve signal, was only a one-way channel. It is now known that the flow of signals, just like a telephone conversation, goes in two directions.[8] And it was once thought that dendrites, those spiderlike endings that arise from the main nerve root, were only receivers of signals. Now it appears that they may leak substances in the opposite direction.[9]

The explosion of knowledge in neurobiology has just begun. New information that humans are learning about their own brains is growing so rapidly that it really does boggle the mind. One of the most important and intriguing findings, however, is that damage to the central nervous system is not necessarily irreparable, as previously maintained, and that critical mental and motor functions may be restored either by

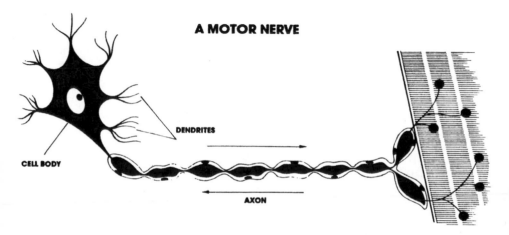

A MOTOR NERVE

DENDRITES

CELL BODY

AXON

nerves forming new connections or shunting signals around injured-tissue roadblocks. *Furthermore, decline in mental function is not an inevitable part of aging.*

The brain is composed of two types of cells, glia (from the Greek word for "glue") and neurons, or nerve cells. Glial cells take care of many of the basic biochemical chores, while neurons perform the main work of the brain, processing impulses from far-flung nerves of the sense organs. Much of this activity is concentrated in the cortex, the thick, folded outer layer of the brain. Groups of neurons on the surface of the cortex process the complex stream of information flowing constantly from the eyes, ears, and other sense organs and nerves throughout the body. The neurons convey these electrical and chemical messages to deeper layers of the cortex and to other underlying brain structures as well as outward to muscles and organs.

Dr. Diamond and her group as well as others have shown, in addition, that glial cells of the brain, which provide support and aid to the neurons, remain in number, even in old age, and are capable of being increased merely by enriching the environment.[10]

In fact, working with mice in the laboratory, Dr. Diamond and her colleagues discovered that an enriched environment could increase the weight of the brain, even in older animals. Dr. Diamond, practicing what she has observed, takes singing lessons to enrich her brain and her life.[11]

Indeed, in long-term studies of humans, it has been shown that people who continue to be active intellectually can actually improve on intelligence tests after the age of sixty.[12]

Working Out Your Brain

Challenging your brain to keep it in optimal condition is vital to not only your central nervous system but to your entire body. Your brain is the most important part of your nervous system—the captain of its organization. For your body to survive, your nervous system must be maintained. All your other organs will undergo sacrifice to keep your brain going when you are under severe stress.

You use only a fraction of your brain's capacity, as pointed out earlier in the foreword. If you don't believe it, consider the fact that people with uncontrollable epilepsy may have as much as half of their brain removed and still function well. In one study of eighty-nine patients who had their frontal lobe of their brain removed, 90 percent were either seizure-free or experienced significant seizure reduction. Five years after surgery, many of the patients were employed full time.[13] And why do some people make a complete recovery from a stroke or serious head trauma? Because other areas of the brain take over for the damaged portion!

Our brains have been designed so well that despite some damage or neglect, we have so much spare capacity that we can often overcome intellectual malfunctions. In fact, the new science of cognitive rehabilitation now being developed to help those whose brains have been severely injured by accidents or strokes has already proven the amazing ability of the brain to overcome deficits by retraining.

THE BRAIN

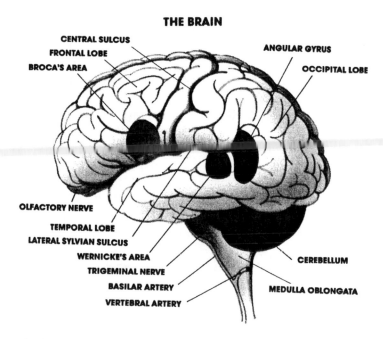

The brain's mastery over even a failing body can be very dramatic. Who was not moved when Kerri Strug, the tiny gymnast in the 1996 Olympics, spectacularly performed her final vault despite an extremely painful injury to her ankle that left her unable to walk after the exhibition was over?

• In a severe and often fatal type of stroke called the Locked-In Syndrome, all four limbs and the speech center of the brain are paralyzed. Some patients recover enough brain function to return to their homes, walk again, and lead fairly normal lives.[14]

• An American tank commander under attack in Vietnam was firing his machine gun when there was a blast next to him. It wasn't until he ran out of ammunition and had to reach down with his left hand to get a new belt that he realized he couldn't use his left hand and that there was something wrong. He was missing a quarter of his brain.[15]

• A forty-four-year-old professor of psychology had a cardiac arrest in which the oxygen was cut off and the right side of his brain was damaged. He awoke in the hospital unable to recall how many children he had. He thought he was ten years younger than he was and he couldn't remember the way to his home. He had to relearn how to play the stereo, set the alarm clock, use a calculator, and change a razor blade. It took him more than seven years, but through a great deal of hard and innovative work, he recovered from his deficits and today is teaching full-time and is in charge of clinical training for graduate psychology students at his former university.[16]

Obviously, recovery from severe brain damage is possible. Intelligence evidently has a lot to do with it. The Vietnam Head Injury Study at Walter Reed Army Medical Center compared post-injury intelligence data with intelligence data obtained from servicemen before they were severely brain injured.[17] The researchers who conducted the massive investigation concluded that a person's "level of experience or intelligence" before a head injury is critical to the recovery of function. The higher the patient's intelligence score before injury, the less likely he is "to show loss" on a post-injury intelligence test. The intelligence factor, they found, is even more important than the size or location of the brain lesion.

Similar findings have been reported in older people. The less educated a person is, the more likely he or she is to develop Alzheimer's disease, according to Claudia Kawas, M.D., an associate professor of neurology at Johns Hopkins Medical Institutions.

"If you are at school when you're young, you may be developing more synaptic connections. It's possible that symptoms of Alzheimer's that occur later are less apparent as a result of this synaptic reserve," Dr. Kawas says. "However, it could be something that correlates with access to education, such as nutritional intake. If you're better educated, you may also more likely be well nourished as a child and this could account for the change in risk."

"Well-educated people may also have more effective strategies for compensating for Alzheimer's disease," Dr. Kawas notes.[18]

We believe, as many researchers do today, that education does not stop in youth; that your brain can benefit from mental exercises. Your brain has a great potential that you have not yet fully tapped. However, the one factor that neuroscientists and psychologists have not been able to measure is personal motivation. This mysterious factor can often be the difference between one patient with severe brain damage making greater progress over another patient with much less damage.

In order to take advantage of this book and the many opportunities available to you today, you must motivate *yourself.*

Those who suffered brain damage within the past few years, such as the psychology professor mentioned earlier, are benefiting from those practicing in the relatively new field of cognitive rehabilitation. Cognitive psychology has borrowed from the techniques developed by experts treating children with learning problems. So, too, we have borrowed techniques from cognitive rehabilitation and the learning disabled that can be adapted to enable healthy people to "brain build." Brain fitness involves motivation, repetition, and "stretching" to improve cognition.

Cognition, by definition, means the process of perceiving or knowing. It includes the following:

- Focusing and sustaining attention
- Differentiating between what is relevant and what is not
- Encoding and storing information—memory
- Organizing and integrating
- Problem solving
- Transmitting and communicating
- Creativity—developing new ways to process and use data

You cannot change your heredity or age just as you cannot change your basic bone structure, but you can use the brain you were given to a greater capacity. Your brain, just like your muscles, will atrophy if not continually exercised.

It has been determined that your brain and peripheral nervous system are like telephone wires that carry conversations back and forth. Specific stimulation will keep your "wires" flowing with the information that initiates the internal and external signals for your thoughts and actions.

It is not too late to start "brain building." Your brain and your nerves are capable of repair and growth in adulthood. In the World Health Organization's *Treatise on Neuroplasticity and Repair in the Central Nervous System,* the general principles state:

> Neuroplasticity does not concern only the recovery of function if this latter is defined as "a return to normal or near-normal levels of performance," following the initially disruptive effects of injury to the nervous system. Neuroplasticity does not refer only to the structural and functional changes of the neuronal organization which follow an injury, but also includes the capacity of the central nervous system to adapt to new physiological conditions emerging either during its maturation or its interaction with the environment. Therefore, neuroplasticity consists of the ability of the nervous system to adapt (in both an anatomical and a functional sense) its structural organization to new situations emerging from developmental and environmental influences as well as from injuries.[19]

Your brain is better designed than any machine on earth and far superior to the brains used by other living creatures. It has the capacity to gather and store an infinite amount of information from without and within and to manipulate that data instantly, not only as it has in the past but in new ways. It is constantly trying to understand itself with finite measurements. Your brain is designed with a lot of area to spare. At any one time, it is estimated you are using 10 percent of your brain. And, like many others, you may abuse your brain by hitting it, bathing it in noxious chemicals, depriving it of necessary nutrients, and allowing it to go "flabby."

In this book, you will read descriptions of exercises for various cognitive functions and some of the theory behind their use. You can use your brain to exercise itself and to "stretch" its own capacity.

2

Sense and Sensitivity: How to Perfect Your Sensory Perception

What happens when you take twenty-two college students and put them into a darkened isolated room where they cannot hear, smell, or see anything, nor can they touch another human being? Within a week, they begin to hallucinate and have peculiar sensory experiences such as smelling something bad or hearing strange sounds.

This is what Dr. Donald Hebb of McGill University, Montreal, Canada, discovered in an experiment performed in the mid-1940s.

His work was followed by that of Dr. John Lilly of the National Institute of Mental Health, Bethesda, Maryland. The American scientist, however, studied the effects of sensory deprivation by immersing his subjects into a tank of tepid water. The volunteers were completely submerged except for a blacked-out head mask through which they breathed. The effect that Dr. Hebb got in several days, Dr. Lilly was able to achieve in a few hours—namely a kind of psychotic-like state from which the subjects recovered as soon as they left the tank and could see, hear, smell, and touch again.[1]

The same phenomena later became apparent to eye doctors and heart specialists. Before the advance of modern technology, patients undergoing cataract surgery to remove the clouded lenses from their eyes were kept in bed, heads immobilized, and both eyes bandaged. Many of the patients—cut off from all visual sensation—suffered dangerous delusional states. They became disoriented, tore at their bandages, and sometimes even attempted suicide. Today eye surgeons operate on only one eye at a time, keep the other eye uncovered, and allow their patients to lead a normal routine, except for bending over.[2]

In the not-too-distant past, heart attack patients were also kept on a regimen of complete rest. To avoid stimulation, the patients were denied radio, television, or visitors. The result was often a condition labeled "cardiac psychosis" in which the patients became irrational and wandered around the ward not knowing where they were. Many physicians at the time believed the state was due to poor circulation, failing heart action, and/or insufficient oxygen to the brain. It was then discovered that heart patients—especially the elderly ones—were suffering from sensory deprivation. Once they were permitted to have music, lights, TV, and visits from relatives, most patients avoided the psychosis and recovered from the heart attack much faster.[3]

Babies and older adults who are not touched suffer not only emotional but physical decline, even to the point of death. We need the stimulation of the touch of others. The manner in which the young of all mammals snuggle and cuddle against the body of the mother and against the bodies of their siblings or of any other introduced animal strongly suggests that cutaneous stimulation is an important biological need for both their physical and their behavioral development.[4] Almost every animal enjoys being stroked. If you own a dog, you know it likes to be petted as long and as often as possible.

Throughout our lives, we humans need our skins caressed and our other senses stimulated. From babies in the crib to old people in nursing homes, we humans need the stimulation and the knowledge gained through our senses to keep our brains functioning well.

What This Means to You

Your brain and nerves have a basic function: to assist you in adapting to perceived changes inside and outside your body. Your nervous system accomplishes this by processing information from your senses.

For example, take an apple in your hand.

Now, how do you know that what you have in your hand is an apple?

First of all, when you took it in your hand, you excited numerous minute sense organs scattered in and below your skin, some of which were particularly sensitive to touch, others to pressure, and yet others to temperature.

The little sense organs sent the fact that you were feeling something cold, round, and smooth to your spinal cord, which in turn relayed the message to your brain.

At the same time, light rays reflected from the surface of the apple stimulating the nerve cells in your eyes. The nerve cells immediately reported back to your brain that you had a red, shiny, round object in your hand.

Still simultaneously, minuscule particles bounding from the apple to the surrounding air excited the tiny nerve cells inside your nose and told your brain how the object in your hand smelled.

Your brain computed all the information you sent it in a time almost too short to calculate, and because it had long ago recorded the fact that a cold, smooth, shiny, round, red, sweet-smelling object is an apple, you realized you had an apple in your hand.

If your brain were to tell you not to eat the apple because it had a worm in it, that would be another story.

This brings us to how you gather information for processing by your brain and how you can maintain and even sharpen your ability to do so.

Any physical change that affects your senses—touch, hearing, sight, smell, and taste—affects your degree of consciousness.

There are your interior perceptions—hunger, thirst, fatigue, heart beat, breathing, and pain. Another perception—that of equilibrium, or balance—tells you of your position in space, right side up or upside down. Still another perception, proprioception, tells you of your activity with the aid of tiny receptors inside your muscles and joints. Most of us aren't even aware we have this muscular sense, yet we use it to determine where in space something is that we are touching and whether it is heavy, light, soft, hard, or gaseous. Here is a simple experiment that illustrates this marvelous, often unheralded sense.

Test Your Proprioception Perception

Take several different-sized cans from your pantry shelf. Place them on the kitchen counter. Now close your eyes and lift each one, and by feel alone place them in descending order of weight. Open your eyes and check your evaluation. How did you know which ones were heavier and which ones were lighter? You used your proprioception sense.

Nerve endings sensitive to movement or pressure are buried in strategic places inside your body. They feed your brain, via your spinal cord, information vital for working your muscles and automatically adjust your limbs and body. They also are involved in the control of your internal organs. Such proprioceptors occur in skeletal and respiratory muscles and are stimulated when the muscle is stretched or shortened. Inside the receptors, which are wound around the striations of the muscles, are specialized fibers containing fine motor nerves; these nerves are believed to be controlled by the cerebellum. Muscles that perform complex, delicate maneuvers, such as those in the fingers and feet, have more spindles per gram of muscle than those that perform less complex movements, like calf muscles.

As we age we may lose some of our proprioceptors, such as those in our joints that react specifically to changes in the angle between two bones. If you have a hip replacement, for example, you can still walk well even though the artificial joint does not have the nerve endings that played a part in your proprioception before replacement. Somehow the body and brain work together to overcome such losses by calling upon other senses, such as vision. It often requires mind over matter—practicing movements to regain control.

Concept of Space/Distance

We also have a mysterious sense of distance or space. In fact, the problem of how any animal locates itself in space is one that has puzzled researchers for a long time. Why can animals follow novel routes to goals? A growing concept today is that an animal has a "brain map" for each environment with which it is familiar. The map may be in the lower center of the brain in an area shaped like a sea horse and given the Greek name for that creature, the *hippocampus*. The "sea horse" is involved in recent memory and behavior. Researchers have discovered that most nerves in the hippocampus fire spatially[5]; that is, an individual nerve cell "lights up" like light bulbs on a marquee. Each cell has its own active region—its spatial field. When they are "turned on" in a certain pattern, they spell out a star's name on a marquee or a location on a brain map. This suggests that the hippocampus is part of a nerve network that informs us just where we are in a particular environment.

Since we can find our way around many different environments, researchers now theorize that hippocampal cells can discriminate between shapes, like rectangles and cylinders. Thus the hippocampal cells are sensitive to the panoramic picture as well as to being "turned on" by a particular shape within the picture.

These findings support the idea that we have environmental space maps in our brains that tell us: What sort of environment we're in, where in this environment we are.[6]

Fingering Space

Shut your eyes and place your hands at your sides. Now, slowly, bring just the tips of your two index fingers together in front of you. Do this four times. How did you know where to touch?

We don't usually exercise our sense of space, because we rely so heavily on our eyes to tell us where we are, but we all have it. As we walk down a dark hallway, for example, we become aware, without touching the wall, that the hallway ends. This may be due to changes in reflected sounds, air pressure, or scent from the walls. The sense of space can be well developed, particularly in blind people.

Finding Your Way with Your Eyes Closed

Choose a blank wall or a closed door. Stand about five feet away from it. Close your eyes and inch your way very slowly toward the wall or door until you believe you are one inch from it. Open your eyes. How accurate were you? You can sharpen your sense of space by periodically closing your eyes and without touching walls or furniture, finding your way along a familiar path, such as the route from your bedroom to your bathroom. Clear away all objects in your path first and, of course, go slowly. Don't try this if you have trouble with your balance. Just imagine that blind people must do this constantly and be precise!

Sensing Time

Still another wonderful sense we use but often do not realize we have is our sense of time.

Short periods of time are difficult to assess unless you count your pulse or notice environmental changes. Longer periods of time can be estimated by observing light changes, hunger sensations, and other body functions, such as the desire to eliminate wastes. Still your sense of time is quite accurate. Test yourself: Look at your watch and observe the time. Now close your eyes. Don't count. Just sit quietly and when you believe three minutes have passed, look at your watch again and check to see how close you were. Do this whenever you are standing in line or waiting in an office for an appointment. It will not only pass the time, it will help sharpen your sense of time.

It is accepted today from studies of the nervous system and behavior that sensory input is critically important for normal development. And yet, none of us fully develops our senses, just as we never use all our brain power, unless circumstances require it.

Helen Keller, for example, who was blind and deaf, could tell a storm's approach before anyone else. She smelled it.

While most of us do not have to concentrate on one sense for information processing as Helen Keller did, we usually favor one sense over another.

A wine connoisseur, for example, can often tell the vineyard in which the wine in a glass was grown and even the year. He or she has a developed sense of taste. A perfumer can walk into your home and identify your cleaning compounds and what you had for dinner the past two nights just by sniffing the air.

An art critic, on the other hand, may look at a few dots of color on a canvas and declare it art worthy of a museum, or a marksman may hit a small moving target at a great distance by looking through a scope. They've both concentrated on their sense of sight. As the great philosopher former Yankee baseball catcher Yogi Berra once said, "You can see a lot just by observing."[7]

Do you love music? It may be those sense organs on the side of your head, your ears, that you favor.

Do you like the feel of velvet? Are you a "toucher"?

Our senses are not only vital for information processing and self-protection, they are the means by which we enjoy living.

One of the fascinating characteristics about perception and sensual pleasure is that it is very brief. Stimulation does not persist with equal response over a period of time. The stimulus must be varied with intervals of rest to remain effective. A popular tune that at first you can't hear often enough will, after prolonged playing, become boring. Eating the same meal, no matter how tasty, will become unappetizing, and thus most people vary their menus.

Fatigue Your Senses

Press your arm against the wall as hard as you can for the count of thirty. Then walk away. Your arm will feel lighter than usual. You have fatigued the nerve cells in your arm and affected how your brain senses it.

Copy the spiral below, punch a hole in the center, and spin it on a pencil point or on a turntable, and stare at it for one minute. Then look at a blank wall or door. What do you see? The spiral will usually go in the opposite direction. This effect is believed to be caused by the tiring of the nerve cells registering movement in the first direction and then the "overflow" firing of the nerve cells detecting movements in the opposite direction.

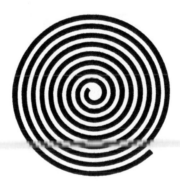

Every sensory experience is appreciated within the context of previous experiences. A child may prefer the most intense new sensory experiences, but when the novelty wears off he becomes bored with it. This search for strong sensation is one of the major reasons some people seek the thrill of psychoactive drugs or unusual sexual exploits. But such a quest is usually endless because the more intense a sensation, the quicker it is gone. On the other hand, if we learn to modulate our senses and develop them even in advanced years, we increase our pleasure in living and we maintain normal function in the cells that receive and respond to sensual input. A decrease in sensory input due to changes in the sense organs or to social isolation is reflected in reduced metabolism and blood flow within the brain.[8] The following information is about the research in progress to understand the interrelationship between our brains and our sense organs. Selective stimulation through conscious effort will enable you to keep the messages flowing that provide you with information about the world around you and the pleasures that give your life meaning.

The Eyes Have It

The sense organs of sight, hearing, touch, taste, and smell report to and are perceived in the cerebral cortex, a huge sheet covering the surface of your brain. It contains as many as ten billion nerve cells—neurons—and the "sheet" is folded to fit inside the skull giving the brain that many-convoluted look. It has been found that a light held above the head evokes nerve cell activity in a different part of the cortex than does a light held below the head. Similarly, a light held directly in front of the viewer activates different parts of the brain's cortex than a light held off to the side. Nerve cells of the visual cortex, the part of the brain to which the eyes report, are highly specialized information-processing machines. It is again similar to light bulbs in a theater marquee. Just as the hippocampal cells "light up" in a certain pattern in response to the environment, the cells of the visual cortex respond to what is seen in a highly specialized manner. Only certain things turn on individual cells.

The Nobel Prize–winning studies of David Hubel and Torsten Wiesel first showed that nerve cells in the cortical area of the brain can be activated only by specific features of what the eyes see.[9] Cortical nerve cells are very often excited more strongly by inputs from one eye than from the other, and Hubel and Wiesel showed that nerve cells that preferred one eye were *clustered* within the cortex and segregated from nerve cells preferring the other eye. Furthermore, the visual brain nerve cells first discovered by Hubel and Wiesel respond best to stimuli of a particular orientation. Some of the visual nerve cells in the brain prefer vertically oriented bars, others horizontally oriented contours, and still others are partial to the oblique. Again, nerve cells that "see" things the same way are clustered together within the brain.

Flashlight Exercises

The purpose of the following flashlight exercises is to stimulate the various areas of your brain involved in light perception.

Take a flashlight, preferably a penlight. Hold it over your head while looking straight ahead; then look up at the light without moving your head. Lower the flashlight to below your chin and, again without moving your head, look down at the light. Count to five and look straight ahead again. Move the flashlight to the right side of your head, about five inches from your ear. Again without moving your head, look to the light, count to five, and look straight ahead. Follow the same steps but switch hands, moving the light to the right side of your head.

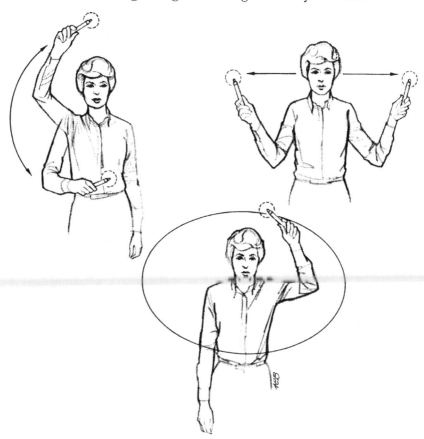

Take the flashlight and, keeping your head motionless, track the flashlight only with your eyes. Move it very slowly in an arc above your head and down below your chin. Then from below your chin to the arc above your head. Repeat five times. Switch hands and repeat.

Now, holding the flashlight, extend your arm out to the side, straight from the shoulder. Pass the flashlight slowly in front of your face at nose level, extending your arm out past the opposite shoulder as far as it will go. Then bring the light slowly back until your arm is at the starting position. Again, track the light only with your eyes. Repeat five times. Put the light in the opposite hand and repeat five times.

Repeat each flashlight exercise with one eye closed. Then repeat with the other eye closed. Do these exercises at least three times a week.

Ball-and-String Exercise

Since research now indicates that the perception of moving objects is most seriously affected by age, stimulating the visual sense is important to driving, flying, or occupations that involve working with moving parts. The following exercise[10] is aimed at this.

Hang a ball (or an empty spool of thread) on a string from above five feet high—it can be from a curtain rod or a chandelier or a branch. Swing the ball as hard as you can, sit down, and track the movement of the ball with your eyes without moving your head or body. Do it for two minutes. Then move your chair to another position, either sideways or on the opposite side of the hanging ball, and repeat, but again, not for more than two minutes. This helps visual tracking, as will watching a tennis match from the sidelines.

Visual Scanning

Visual scanning is necessary for many activities, such as accurately perceiving and locating objects in space, operating a car, and working machinery. Crossword and jigsaw puzzles are excellent for scanning and thinking. The following is an exercise used to demonstrate your ability to scan.

Find and cross out the letter S wherever you find it in the box below within 30 seconds.

```
X E D C F S G H J S E T Y X S D Q P O L L G M N B T H H M A S X C V
S E W Q C B G S T N S P O L R T Y U N B F E R W S T Y U J H G B V C
W X C Q A T Y U S D C V H S K L P O B N I Y T H G S F V C B Z A R T
X E R T Y V B D S F E X L K S R U O N M E R S D Q T C V B Y Q P L K
P Z W E Q S C G T S B T B H U I O P L J S D C B T Y H F G K J L S M
O W S Q T Y U K J H G S C V B N M T H S J L W S L F V B T H S N M W
C B V N M J H S D F G H T Y S V C X S B R T C D S T U Y T N M K R S
B D F T R S D U I K L U Y T R P B S C V T E W X Z A Q W S B K I T Y
```

When you are waiting in a doctor's office or a beauty salon or barber shop, you can take a pencil and cross out a single letter on a printed page in a magazine, for example. It's good exercise, if the owner doesn't mind.

Visual-Spatial Orientation

This is a skill needed for identifying and perceiving objects with different forms in various positions. Circle the objects that are alike in this illustration.

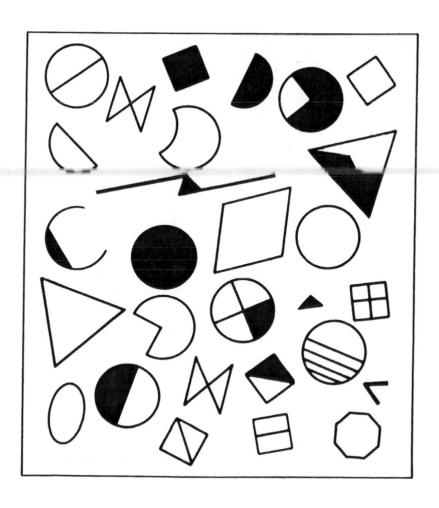

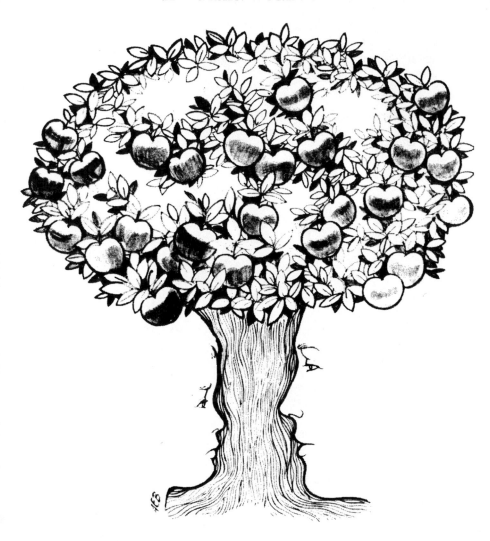

Can You Believe Your Eyes?

When you look at the picture above, what do you see? An apple tree or a mother and child? Your brain perceives only one image at a time, so your perception may shift back and forth. You may also see something in a picture that another does not see. The famed ink blot or Rorschach test is an example, in which psychotherapists interpret what a person perceives in an irregular stain.

Ignore the "Noise"

Being able to perceive despite background "noise" is an ability that can be improved. For example, look at the following geometric forms and find the designated one in the larger boxes to the right.

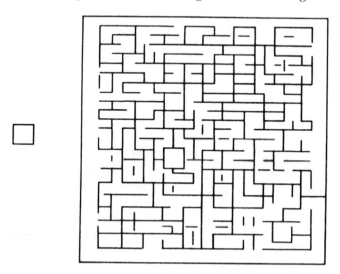

Find and circle the square within four seconds.

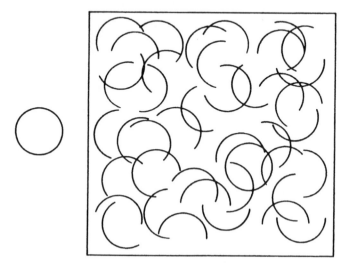

Find and circle the circle within three seconds.

Let There Be Light

Metabolism refers to the chemical processes through which your body changes air, food, and other materials into substances it needs to function properly. The rate at which your metabolism functions may be different from those of other people. It is determined by the genes you inherit and other factors, such as what you eat and the time of day. How you expose yourself to light can greatly affect your metabolism, as well as your mood and behavior. Light involves intensity, spectrum, and timing.

It has recently been acknowledged that humans, like other animals, can have their hormones manipulated by changing light. The pineal gland in the brain, for example, normally releases its hormone, *melatonin*, at night and shuts down during the day.

The duration of melatonin secretion depends on the duration of the darkness; hence, twenty-four-hour melatonin secretion is greater during the winter than during the summer. Exposure to light at night inhibits melatonin secretion in a dose-dependent fashion; the brighter the light, the greater the decrease in plasma melatonin concentration. On the other hand, exposure to darkness during the day does not increase melatonin emission.

At the time and immediately after a change to night-shift work or travel across time zones, melatonin output is desynchronized and contributes to that hangoverlike fatigue we call "jet lag."

In 1980 Dr. Alfred Lewy, a research psychiatrist then at the National Institute of Mental Health, showed that the release of human melatonin can be blocked by light at least ten times brighter than ordinary room light.[11] He showed that exposure to very bright lights in the visible spectrum during the normally dark parts of a person's day could suppress the release of melatonin. He also demonstrated the ability of very bright light in the morning and evening to bring dramatic relief to patients who suffer severe winter-long depressions. You can use light to raise your spirits and to improve your visual perceptions.

• Use a 250-watt bulb in your reading lamps. But the best reading light is still natural light from a window. It is brighter and more diffuse, equal to about 5,000 candles.

• Sit closer to the light, within two feet.

• Fluorescent light is very good. It is diffuse and cooler and doesn't create a glare.

• When weather permits, open your window. Ordinary window glass filters out ultraviolet rays. In the winter, spend more time outdoors in the middle of the day, when the light is brightest, for example, by walking to your lunch appointment.

The Sense of Hearing—Have You Heard About It?

Remember that old nursery rhyme:

> *Here was an old owl liv'd in an oak*
> *The more he heard, the less he spoke*
> *The less he spoke, the more he heard*
> *O, if men were like that wise bird.*

Next to vision, hearing is probably the sense most used to gather information (although some people do have difficulty really listening because they're always talking).

Almost all the thousands of single tones processed by the human ear are heard by a mechanism known as *air conduction.* In this process, sound waves are first funneled through the externally visible part of the ear and the *external auditory canal* to the *ear drum*, which vibrates at different speeds. The *hammer* (malleus), which is attached to the tympanic membrane, transmits the vibrations to the *anvil* (incus). The vibrations then pass on to the *stirrup* (stapes) and *oval window* to the inner ear. In the inner ear, the fluid-filled spiral passage of the *snail* (cochlea) contains cells whose microscopic hairs respond to the vibrations produced by sound. The hair cells, in turn, excite the 28,000 fibers of the auditory nerve that end in the middle of your brain. Auditory information flows via the *thalamus* to the *temporal gyrus,* the part of the brain involved in receiving and perceiving sound.

The physiology of the sense of hearing is quite easily measured since the brain and body are so responsive to sounds. Pleasant auditory stimulation—music, for example—can produce both emotional and physical benefits. One of the reasons that music affects us physically is that it has rhythm (called *pulse*) and tempo *(pace),* and so do we. The continuous beat of our heart is the most fundamental of all musical rhythms; listen to a primitive drumbeat, for example, and you'll hear a beating heart. Listen to disco music and you'll hear it again. The pulsing beat so closely matches our own heart rate that we feel an urge to move our body in sync with the music. Music can calm and excite our emotions, raise or lower our blood pressure, affect our respiration and brain cells. It can also destroy our hearing mechanism if played too loudly.[12]

In general, a decibel represents the difference the human ear can detect between the loudness of two sounds. Conversation in a relatively quiet setting ranges around 60 decibels, and the roar of traffic or sounds of factory machinery are typically about 80 decibels. Anything above 80 is uncomfortable, and at 90, the experts start worrying about the effects on health. A food blender, for example, is 93 decibels, and a reving motorcycle, 110. Loud noise and noise that may be soft but irritating can produce harmful effects physically and mentally.[13] If you doubt the effect of sound on your body, just consider how you felt when someone slammed a door unexpectedly or a teacher scratched chalk on the blackboard.

Hearing loss, however, is one of the most difficult sensory losses to tolerate since it affects verbal communication, essential for social and environmental well-being. The stress of not hearing well also causes mental irritation and, at times, withdrawal and depression.

Fifty percent of those over age sixty-five suffer from some form of hearing impairment. This problem usually begins at about age twenty and has been estimated to affect as many as 66 percent of the people over age eighty.

Loss of hearing is not a normal part of aging. In less industrialized, quieter societies, hearing is as keen at seventy-five years as it is at seventeen years.[14] It has been reported a number of times that the popularity of loud rock-and-roll music has resulted in significant loss of hearing in many young people. It is most unwise for anyone to have music blasting through headphones, a common custom today. It can be not only painful, but cause permanent effects on your ability to hear and understand.

Sounds follow two paths to the brain; one to the auditory center on the side of the brain, where it is perceived and interpreted, and the other to the base of the brain, where the control center for the autonomic nervous system lies. The autonomic nervous system involves the functions of the respiratory, circulatory, digestive, and urogenital systems, as well as the action of glands and the involuntary muscles in the skin. Just remember how you feel when a loud noise startles you. Your heart beats faster, you catch your breath and your stomach knots. That would be a strong response to a startling noise, but even sounds to which you have become habituated and relatively oblivious may still provoke a physical fight-or-flight response—an increase in heart rate and blood pressure, constriction of the small blood vessels in the extremities, and release of the stress-related adrenal hormones. The auditory system does have an effect on the frontal lobe, which is involved in personality and intellectual function. Failure in the auditory pathways is believed by some to be the core defect in schizophrenia.

Scientists are studying how the brain "hears" by use of *evoked potentials,* measurements of the electrical output of the brain (EEG) in response to a stimulus. It is an electrical measurement like voltage in an electrical line. Signal transmission is called the *potential.* To measure the current, a stimulus must be used to "evoke" it, such as a click or flashing light.

A fraction of a second after a person hears a click, for example, electrodes on the scalp can begin detecting the transmission of the "sound" from the ear, through the brain stem, and into the upper brain. The first component of the tracing is generated near the inner ear; components two through five arise in different regions of the brain stem. Where the signals go after that is still controversial, but it is known that by the time ten milliseconds have elapsed, the electrical response has probably reached the cerebral cortex, the "thinking brain."

In experiments at the University of Maryland, researchers played tones into the right ears of subjects and evoked an electrical brain-signal response on the right side of their brains. When, however, the researchers again played the tone into the subjects' right ears but asked the subjects to count the tones in the left ear, the evoked electrical activity appeared on left side of the brain.

While this work is far from completely accepted, it seems to show that consciously making an effort to identify various stimuli can stimulate different areas of the brain.

In the meantime, it is up to you to protect your hearing by avoiding loud and/or irritating noise and by having any ear infections treated promptly. If you have to constantly say "What? What?" to people, have your hearing tested. There is no shame in augmenting your hearing with an aid, no more than there is to improving your vision with glasses.

The following are a few exercises for those hearing centers in your brain.

Talk Like the Animals

You'll probably want to do this while no one is around or with someone who wants to perform, too. Imitate as many animal sounds as you can—dog, cat, tiger, coyote, bird, and so on into a tape recorder. The next day, play back the tape and try to identify the animals you were imitating. Then make another tape, this time imitation of common noises in your environment, such as your car, the telephone, the door bell, and repeat the procedures.

Music and Mood

Music—pleasant sounds—can have a profound effect on mood, as we have pointed out.

Leo Shatin, Ph.D., former professor of clinical psychology at Mount Sinai School of Medicine in New York City and a researcher in music psychology, tested the mood-altering effects of music in a group-therapy setting: "We found that with slow, sad music people interacted less frequently. When someone finally did speak, it was usually with anger or hostility. Upbeat, cheerful songs, on the other hand, had people talking more and in a more friendly way."[15]

Mood altering through music seems quite logical, according to Shelley Katsh, a certified music therapist. The theory: Certain musical abilities—singing, for example—are thought to be located in the same side of the brain, the right, as are our feelings and emotions.

Find That Beat

Go over your tapes or CDs and choose a happy, fast-paced song; a slow, quiet one; and a moody, melancholy one.

Now, identify your mood. Are you agitated and nervous? If so, start out with the fast-paced music, the "jumping sound," and gradually change the CD or tape until you have serene, calm music playing.

Are you depressed or sluggish? Start with the slow, moody music and gradually change to light, happy music. You'll be surprised at how the music changes your mood. Here are some other tips:

• Do not listen to music for more than twenty minutes at a time, because it can fatigue your senses.

• Do not listen to music while you are trying to do a difficult intellectual task. It will interfere.

• Use music to lull you to sleep.

- Use music to create a romantic interlude. Usually, the music that was popular during the teenage years of the one you are trying to put in a romantic mood is the music to play.

Hear the News?—Increase Your Perception

Just as you can train your muscles to perform better, so, too, you can increase your auditory perception.

Get a news program or talk show on your radio, and turn the volume all the way down. Then draw a straight line on a piece of paper with your dominant hand.

Place the point of your pencil at the beginning of the line. With your nondominant hand, slowly turn the volume up at the same time that you very, very slowly move the point of the pencil along the line. As soon as you can understand what is being said on the radio, make a mark on the line.

Keep repeating the process, trying to make the mark on the line earlier each time. (Try hard to turn up the radio volume and draw the line at approximately the same speed each time you repeat the exercise.) This exercise is aimed at sharpening your hearing and your concentration. It would be beneficial to do it every day, but it should be done at least once a week.

Protect Your Brain Against Dangerous Noise

Unpleasant sound to you, personally, is noise. It can be annoying and affect your mood. It may also be dangerous to your hearing. You know noise is potentially harmful if:

- you have to shout over background noise to make yourself heard;
- the noise hurts your ears or makes your ears ring;
- you are slightly deaf for several hours after exposure to the noise.

How to judge sound levels in decibels:

- Quiet library, soft whisper 30 decibels
- Heavy city traffic, alarm clock at two feet 80 decibels
- Chain saw, boiler shop or pneumatic drill 100 decibels

(Exposure for more than two hours may damage your hearing.)

- Rock concert in front of speakers, thunderclap, gun fire 120 decibels

(May cause immediate ear injury.)

Noise may not be loud enough to damage your sense of hearing but unwanted sound can cause a lot of problems for your sense of well-being. Annoying noise is a personal thing; what bothers you may sound like music to someone else. If you are subjected constantly to unwanted sound, from someone's snoring or a gardener's leaf blowing, you can suffer anxiety, depression, sleeplessness, and other health problems. Here are some suggestions you can use to ease chronic noise problems.

• Carpeting can absorb more than half of all airborne noises. Upholstered furniture also soaks up sound, as do pillows.

• Curtains and draperies keep things more quiet by sound absorption. Covering walls with well-filled bookcases has a similar effect. If necessary, the ceilings of your home can be covered with acoustical tile, which can absorb up to 75 percent of excess noise.

• Windows can now be purchased that are especially made to screen out noise.

• Inexpensive weather stripping can be used to stop noise from entering through gaps in doors and windows.

• Dishwashers or washing machines that cause sound pollution can be mounted on felt, cork, or rubber to absorb vibrations. Make sure the appliances are level on the floor.

• Distance is one of the least expensive methods for controlling noise.

• "Acoustical perfume"—recordings of pleasant sounds—can be used to cover unpleasant noise, much as deodorants are used to mask bad odors.

• Failing all else, use of inexpensive earplugs or ear protects may be the only solution.

The Sweet Smell of Stimulation

Gourmets may be proud of their sense of taste, yet taste is mostly smell. The senses of smell and taste are inextricably connected.

Our sense of taste is powerful. We can identify quinine, for instance, in as little as a one-part-per-billion solution, but taste pales next to our amazing ability to smell. We can detect an unlimited number of odors, some from far away and in dilutions as weak as one part in several billion parts of air. Nomads supposedly can smell a campfire thirty miles across a breezeless desert.

Everything has an odor to some degree, but particles for either taste or smell must be soluble. This is a throwback to our ancestral life in the sea when smell and taste were one. Sugar has no taste on a dry tongue, just as the scent of roses would go unnoticed in a dry nose.

The importance of each sense varies with each species. Birds, for instance, are said to rely very little on olfaction and depend mainly on sight and sound, while insects and the majority of mammals are dependent on their sense of smell. Until recently, humans were reluctant to admit they were affected physiologically and psychologically by what they smelled.

In 1959 researchers coined the word *pheromone*—from the Greek *pherein* meaning "to carry" and *horman* meaning "to excite or stimulate"—to describe certain substances produced by the glands of animals. *Hormones*, the secretions of glands, also are named from *horman* because they "arouse to action." The difference between pheromones and hormones is that hormones are secreted by an animal's own glands into its own bloodstream and affect the animal's own body and behavior. Pheromones, on the other hand, are also secreted by an animal's glands but are carried through the air to affect the body and behavior of another animal. You only have to have the experience of owning a female cat or dog in heat to know the power of pheromones. Male animals from near and far will arrive at your door, frenzied by the female scent.

Though we may wish to deny it, we humans are manipulated by smells just as the butterfly, the salmon, and the ape are. There are many scientists who now maintain that we emanate sexual scents and that "love at first sight" is really "love at first scent."

Our human olfactory cells are identical in construction to those of all other creatures, from one end of the animal kingdom to the other. And while we may not be as good at smelling as the bloodhound or the shark, our normal sense of smell is pretty remarkable, and when fully developed, it is astounding. One society matron, who wished to remain anonymous, amazed scientists in the 1940s with her ability to identify smells. She could report who last slept on a newly laundered pillowcase and was able to match coats in a closet to guests at a party by scent alone.

When we smell a perfume or baking bread, we smell the molecules of scent that have drifted to our noses. The odor molecules are inhaled with the air and dissolved on the wet film of mucus in our noses. Information about the molecules is relayed by sensory cells high in each nasal passage to the olfactory bulb, where it is sent along tracts in the olfactory lobe to the brain. We then realize within a thousandth of a second that the person is wearing a particular scent. But how is the message encoded and delivered to the brain? How does the nose select one molecule over another, enabling one scent to overcome another? Why is the filing system of scent memories so efficient and apparently indestructible that we never forget what we have smelled, once the scent has been identified.[16]

The incredibly specialized odor sensory cells, located high in an inaccessible place at the top of each nasal passage, are pigmented yellow or brownish yellow, which distinguishes them from the ordinary cells of the nose. In humans they occupy an area about the size of a dime, whereas the smell sensory area in a dog or rabbit is about the size of a handkerchief.

Neuroanatomists have found the olfactory system unique because instead of going through the thalamus—that large area of brain just above the brain stem that acts as a relay station for the other senses to the neocortex, that "new" part of the brain that gives us our intellect—the olfactory cells send their fibers directly to the brain area formerly called the rhinencephalon (from the Greek for "nose brain"). At one time this area—which is considered the oldest in evolutionary terms—was believed to deal only with smell, hence the name. More than thirty years ago, however, anatomists found that this so-called nose brain also deals with the regulation of motor activities and the primitive drives of sex, hunger, and thirst. Therefore, the term *rhinencephalon* was changed to *limbic system*, derived from the limbus, or border, rimming the cortex of the brain.

The construction of these cells is similar in all mammals, including humans. Each of the cells has cilia on its exposed side, and on the inside, there are nerve endings that lead directly to one of the two olfactory bulbs of the brain, through the sievelike openings of the ethmoid bone located behind the bridge of the nose. The two olfactory bulbs are beneath the brain's frontal lobes.

Stimulation of the olfactory bulb shoots electrical signals to an almond-shaped area known as the *amygdala*. This area of the limbic system is concerned with visceral and behavioral mechanisms, particularly those associated with sensory and sexual functions. These signals are then relayed from the amygdala to the brain stem, the "turnpike" that contains the interconnections between brain and body. Therefore, the electrical stimulation involved in smelling directly affects the digestive and sexual systems and emotional behavior. Destruction of the amygdala area has resulted in a loss of fear and rage reactions, an increase in sexual activity, excessive eating, and severe deficiencies in memory.[17]

In 1937 Japanese researchers first reported there was electrical activity in sensory cells of the nose and in the brain when an odor stimulus occurred. It was not until the 1940s and 1950s that such electrical pulses were measured systematically as to strength, duration, and quality. The brain's electrical response to an odor—about forty cycles per second—appears to be indistinguishable from that correlated with emotional behavior. Since olfactory signals are sent to the amygdala area, it is easy to explain how what we smell affects our emotions and our sex and hunger drives.

A U.S. company, the Pherin Corporation, is aiming to develop pharmaceuticals that will use the chemical-sensitive receptors in the nose that are directly linked by nerves to the hypothalamus in the brain, a region involved in emotions, sex drive, water and salt balance, and blood pressure. The company, which calls the family of medications *vomeropherins*, notes that the compounds can be applied to the nose to affect brain function without entering blood circulation. They are expected to act rapidly with a low side-effect potential and to only affect specific regions of the brain. One class of their compounds, the corporation reports, seems to counteract anxiety. A second group evoked changes in specific hormone levels.

Since scents affect our emotions, and may also attract us to a potential mate, pharmaceuticals through the nose seem very logical. There are many conflicting opinions among researchers as to how the brain identifies smells, however. Some maintain that the olfactory bulb has been mapped for specific odors. For example, the inhalation of fruity odors activates the front part of the bulb, while solvents such as benzene stimulate preferentially the back part of the bulb. Until quite recently, scientists did not know that the trigeminal nerve in the cheek is involved in mediating certain chemical sensitivities to smells. The trigeminal receptors—which are bare nerve endings dispersed in the nasal passageway, mouth, throat, and in mucosa around the eyes—communicate with the brain via the cheek's trigeminal nerve. In principle, the odor can be sensed through the interaction with either of these receptors or the smell sensory cells or with both.

A unique and as yet unexplained phenomenon of smell is that of adaptation. You know that no matter how strong an odor is when you enter a room, you become unaware of it or blind to it after a few minutes. When subjects are tested for recognition of certain odors, there has to be a pause of at least thirty to sixty seconds between stimulations before any odor, new or the same, can be recognized. It has also been shown that prior exposure to one odorant will decrease the sensitivity to another. A higher concentration of the second odor is therefore required for detection.

When scientists record the electrical activity that smelling an odor causes in the olfactory bulb, they find that even though the subjects can no longer detect the odor—say, of pine—the electrical signals continue unabated in their brains. In other words, the physical stimulus— the pine odor—still is at work but the subject is no longer aware of the scent.

Why is there adaptation? No one knows for certain, but some theorize that it is somehow involved in the protection of respiration. Perhaps we would stop breathing, or be unable to concentrate, or our other senses would become overpowered by our concentration on odor if we were constantly aware of a particular scent.

We influence our own behavior and the behavior of others with both natural and synthetic smells, often subconsciously. More and more research is taking place trying to understand this link between odors and behaviors. It is obvious that reactions to a specific smell are spontaneous and immediate. The sudden appearance of an odor can cause measurable changes in the resistance of the skin of a person quite similar to that which takes place if he or she is suddenly startled.

When an odor is liked there is a relaxation of the facial muscles, smiling, a pleasant tone of voice, laughing, nodding, opening of the mouth, and deeper respiration. When an odor is disliked, there is a turning away of the head and sometimes the entire body. The head may be jerked back, the nose wrinkled and the upper lips raised.

Association with experience may play a part in determining such reactions, since odors are so closely linked to emotions and memory. Coloring may also affect the sense of pleasantness and unpleasantness. Green coffee would not smell as good as brown, and black strawberries would not seem as fragrant as red.

Manufacturers have made "new car smells" to make us think better of a used car, and the scent of bread baking is deliberately wafted into the street so that pedestrians will be enticed into a bakery. Using the scent of flowers to cover our own human scents is a multibillion-dollar industry. We are all led around by our noses. A British company has even come up with an olfactory "security blanket." Named Osmone 1, it consists of a sandalwood-like blend of mammary and armpit scents, which supposedly mimics a newborn's smell of mother, triggering a secure feeling in adults.

Smell tells us about the chemical nature of things. Harmful things usually smell bad, but not always. Good things usually smell good, but not always. Some things smell good at one time and bad at others. Have you ever smelled food cooking when you were nauseated?

Furthermore, smells that may be pleasant or appropriate for one place may be unpleasant or inappropriate for another. Would you want to eat in a restaurant that smells like a dentist's office? On the other hand, would you let a dentist work on your mouth if his office smelled like a restaurant?

Our principal objective in attempting to get rid of an odor is most often to avoid giving offense to others. We do not want to be embarrassed. Bad odors make us uncomfortable—even sick.

On the other hand, our ability to smell a bad odor can protect us. Without it, we may be overcome by gas or by rotten food. Therefore, we must do everything to keep our sense of smell in as sharp a condition as possible.

Importance of the Sense of Smell

As people get older, they may not be able to detect odors as well as they could in the past. The sense of smell may also be lost due to sinus or nasal disease, medication, or gum diseases, all of which are treatable. However, the loss of smell due to a virus or a head injury has not as yet been able to be restored.

It is important to sharpen the sense of smell when possible.

Making Scent Associations

Take a pad and pencil and write down in a column your four favorite smells. Now write down your four most disliked smells.

Next to each smell, write your associations with those smells. If baking associates baking bread with the warmth of your mother's kitchen on Sunday morning, smelling baking bread should bring that image to mind. Then write down whatever you associate with the bad smells and compare with your favorite smells.

After you have completed the list and associations, read it. It will give you a great deal of insight into your emotional history and will have stimulated that area of the brain involved with odor and emotions.

Stimulate Your Olfactory Nerves

Take six envelopes and six cotton swabs and six small pieces of paper. Dip a swab—so that you get just a tiny drop of the liquid on it—in vanilla. Write down "vanilla" on the piece of paper and slip the swab and the paper in an envelope.

Repeat the procedures with a swab dipped in ammonia cleaner, a cooking oil, water, alcohol, and vinegar.

Once the swabs with their identifications are in the envelopes, shuffle them.

Close your eyes, remove each swab, and sniff. (Allow a count of sixty between sniffs.) Write down the identification of scent in the order you sniffed them. Your best memory is your odor memory. Just by testing it, you are using the olfactory lobe of your brain.

Odors, as we have pointed out, have a great deal to do with emotions and behavior. Susan Schiffman, Ph.D., of Duke University, a researcher in olfaction, maintains that women in their twenties use odor to attract; in their thirties, to define their territory; in their fifties, as an antidepressant; and in their sixties, as a stimulus.[18]

You can change your mood with pleasant scents. Oriental perfumes are sultry and sexy; fruity, classic florals and green blends are reminiscent of the garden; and woodsy or leather scents are thought to be masculine. Herbal is popular among those who want to feel healthy and clean, as they contain a medicinal or phenolic note.

To stimulate your sense of smell, imitate the Greeks who brought the scent of nature indoors. The Greeks had living rooms that opened onto beautiful gardens, where the most fragrant plants were placed near the windows in the belief that the scent had a salutary effect on the occupants of the house. In medieval monasteries, also, the monks planted sweet-smelling herbs near infirmaries for the benefit of their patients.

Those lucky enough to have gardens should consider the scenting of their homes when planting them. Night-blooming flowers can be placed by bedroom windows and day-blooming plants by the kitchen and living room windows.

Those who live in apartments can bring all sorts of fragrant plants into their homes, which not only beautify but humidify, deodorize, and scent the air with their leaves and blooms.

Lavender has been used for centuries on sheets to encourage peaceful sleep, and rooms scented with roses have been used as a tranquilizer.

A Matter of Taste

If everything tasted alike, eating would be boring. Flavor is a combination of taste and smell, yet according to Israeli scientists, these two perceptions go to different parts of the brain. Weizmann Institute researchers Professor Yadin Dudai and graduate student Rina Schul and Professor Burton Slotnick of the American University in Washington, D.C., found that taste qualities are probably stored in or around the gustatory cortex in the brain's upper-rear lobe, while smell is delivered to a lower olfactory area in the brain. Yet nerve signals conveying taste and smell converge in the brain's frontal lobe—the motor area responsible for instructions of movement and speech. The frontal lobe also is home to faculties of planning and mental representation of the outside world.

The two senses together allow us to distinguish thousands of different flavors. Alone, taste is a relatively primitive sense. This combination explains why loss of the sense of smell also apparently causes a serious reduction in taste.

The Israeli researchers also found that during the creation of a taste memory, an atom of phosphorus is added to various nerve cell proteins—creating a molecular "memo." They believe the new understanding of how long-term taste memory is stored will be applicable to understanding how other memories are stored and will lead to medications to strengthen or weaken people's memories.[19]

Taste gives us great pleasure and at the same time protects us from bad food. For the most part, that which is good for us is pleasant tasting and that which is bad is awful in our mouth. The mouth is the first part of our digestive tracts. Our teeth crush food so that enzymes can break it down, while saliva lubricates it to make it easier to swallow.

Our tongues have a complex system of muscles that enables them to move food around as we chew, and then to mold chewed food into a ball for swallowing. The surface of our tongues is covered with minute hairlike projections surrounded by tastebuds.

The tastebuds can distinguish four main types of flavor: sweet, salt, sour, and bitter. Tastebuds were designed to warn you about rotten food and to give you pleasure so that you wouldn't forget to eat. There is a preference for sweetness at birth, but there is a difference, perhaps genetic, perhaps learned, in the levels of sweetness as we mature.

The front of the tongue is the most convenient and most widely used for taste testing because it is readily accessible and contains very few sensory fibers other than taste.

Tastebuds do diminish as most people age. At age seventy, the average person has fewer taste buds than at age thirty. Most researchers agree that all four basic tastes commonly decline: sweet, salty, and bitter usually after fifty years; sour after sixty years.[20]

The lips are involved in not only processing food and drink for taste and nourishment, but also are important to our sense of touch. Why else would we kiss? By stimulating the nerve endings on your lips and tongue, you stimulate the brain areas that receive their messages. Stimulation of the senses, as we have pointed out, helps preserve and improve function and increase pleasure.

Lip Exercises—Puckers and Smiles
   • Rip a piece of paper into inch-long shreds and scatter the pieces on a tabletop. Place a saucer and a straw on the tabletop. Pick up each piece of paper by sucking it up with the straw and holding it by suction until you can transfer it to the saucer.
   • Take a cotton ball and blow it across a table.
   • Practice sounding out *U, P, B, M, D, W.*
   • Whistle a happy tune.
   • Tuck in your lips over your teeth and grin.
   • Relax your lips and then move them toward one ear and then toward the other.
   • Smile as hard as you can.
   • Alternate pursing and retracting your lips.
   • Stick out your tongue as far as you can and then wag it from side to side.
   • Lick your tongue all around your lips as if you ate something absolutely delicious.

THE TONGUE—A MAP OF TASTE BUDS

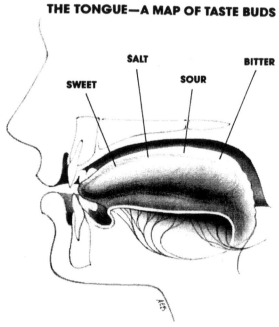

Taste Exercise

Take five envelopes and five cotton swabs and dip one swab in salt, another in lemon, another in sugar, another in vinegar, and the last in water.

Place the swabs in envelopes with their identifications written on small pieces of paper. Close your eyes.

With one hand, gently touch the top of your tongue with a swab and try to identify the taste. Repeat with the left rear side of your tongue and the right rear side. Write down what you believe the taste is. Wait sixty seconds and repeat with another swab. Repeat the tasting procedure for each swab.

Check your answers against the slips of paper in the envelopes.

Do this at least once a month, preferably once a week, with a variety of taste samples of your choice.

Restaurant Guesser

To sharpen your perception of taste, try to guess the spices used in a particular restaurant dish. Write them down on a piece of paper and ask your server to take the paper to the chef to see how accurate you are. The chef may be flattered.

Touch Me in the Morning

The surface of the skin has an enormous number of sensory receptors receiving stimuli of heat, cold, touch, and pain. It is estimated that there are some fifty receptors per one hundred square millimeters. The number of tactile points varies from 7 to 135 per square centimeter. There are more than a million sensory fibers from the skin entering the spinal cord.

The continuous stimulation of the skin by the external environment serves to maintain both sensory and motor tonus. The brain must receive sensory feedback from the skin in order to make such adjustments as may be called for in response to the information it receives. If your arm goes to sleep while you are lying on it, your skin will tell your brain to "move it."

Touching is perhaps our swiftest and most direct form of communication. When you touch people, their skin surfaces have millions of sensory receptors that inform them about not only heat, cold, and pain, but literally how you feel about them.

Touch is a form of nonverbal communication that has been neglected compared to other kinds of expression. One reason that it has not been studied as much is that it borders on being a taboo subject. How and with whom you touch is carefully controlled, especially in this day and age when an innocent touch may be considered "sexual harassment" or "molestation." Yet you rarely go through the day without being touched or touching someone.

We use touch to describe our feelings and our other sensations. If a patient has a chest pain and presses his chest with a clenched fist, this usually signifies that the pain is widespread and has a gripping quality. The pain from peptic ulcer is often closely localized, and the patient usually tells a doctor so by delicately pointing to it with the tip of the index finger. If the pain is more or less superficial—what would normaly be called soreness—the patient may lightly brush the surface of the skin with the outstretched tips of all five fingers.

The brain has a very large area reserved to receive messages from the various sensors in the skin. Nerve fibers conducting tactile impulses are generally of larger size than those associated with the other senses. In fact, human beings can lose their organs of sight, hearing, smell, and taste, but they cannot lose their skin and survive.

Touch Language

We can reach out and touch someone or we can draw back. We can slap when we are angry and caress when we are loving. Such gestures are obvious, but you can also practice "reading" through your skin. Have someone lightly draw numbers or letters or even words on your back with a finger or pencil, and try to identify the message. Different areas of the body vary in their sensitivity to touch discrimination and painful stimuli according to the number and distribution of receptors. The cornea is several hundred times more sensitive to painful stimuli than are the soles of the feet. The fingertips are good at touch discrimination but the chest and back are less sensitive.

Have You Hugged Your Pillow Today?

You can reach out and touch someone or some animal. If you are too shy or do not have a pet to stroke, then adopt the Chinese custom. Buy a soft bolster, an elongated pillow, or just a large bed pillow. Almost everybody in China, including males, is given pillows from the time of birth. These pillows for holding are small for infants, larger for older children, and the largest size is for adults. You can wrap your arms and legs around them. They are soft and filled with cotton and cuddly. Even in the Chinese bridal chamber, the bed is furnished with a bolster, just one, placed in the middle of the bed.

Take a pillow to bed with you and cuddle it. The feeling of comfort you will receive will probably be due to your brain's release of its own tranquilizers, the endorphins, in response to the stimulation of your skin by your hugging of the pillow.

The Massage Is the Message

Many cultures have recognized that the "laying on" of hands is healing, relaxing, and sensual. If you have someone who will massage your skin with a favorite lotion, that is ideal. If not, you can be nice to yourself. Starting at your toes, and working your way up your body, including your arms and neck, to your face, massage gently, with or without lotion, while you are relaxed. Soft music and a darkened room may help. Have a massage at least once a week, or more often if you are very tense or feeling "blue." Again, the stimulation your brain receives from stroking the skin is soothing because your brain responds to it by releasing its tranquilizing endorphins.

Touch Identification

Gather a variety of materials, such as a swatch of terry cloth, a piece of velvet, cotton balls, feathers, and sandpaper. Put one of each material in an unmarked envelope. Shuffle the envelopes. Close your eyes and, with just the tip of your index finger, feel the material and write the identification down. If you have another person available, lie on your abdomen and have your partner lightly rub each material against your bare back while you try to identify it.

Some Like It Hot, Not Too Hot

The upper limit of tolerable body temperatures in most land vertebrates is 104° to 122°F (40° to 50°C). Although excessive temperatures affect virtually every organ, the brain function appears to be especially vulnerable to heat. If the brain is kept cool, tolerance to elevated body temperature is extended. The temperature of the mammalian brain is determined by the rate of heat production of brain cells, the rate of blood flow through the brain, and the temperature of the blood supplying the brain. In addition, the temperature of the surface regions of the brain can be influenced by direct heat exchange through the scalp or through the base of the skull. We cool ourselves by sweating on the face. Fanning the face causes the temperature of the brain to drop.

Temperature affects how well we think. The cognitive performance of six male Marines undergoing a heat-acclimatization regimen was assessed using repeated learning and time-estimation tasks. Subjects performed controlled treadmill exercises in a heat-acclimatization chamber at 33.3°F (4°C). Their performance was tested several times during the 155 minutes that they were exposed to heat. On the first day of heat exposure, their ability to accurately estimate time fell below the level of that demonstrated in the same exercise at moderate room temperature, as did their capacity to learn. By the tenth day of heat exposure, all subjects demonstrated significant heat acclimatization. However, their learning tasks were still impaired and their time estimates were higher than during the first heat exposure. These results suggest that learning new tasks may be difficult in a hot environment, even for partially acclimatized individuals.[21]

Temperature Test Yourself

This exercise requires a home thermostat. Try to memorize passages from a book at 65°F (18.33°C); 70°F (21.11°C); 78°F (25.55°C). Choose the temperature at which learning was easiest. It would be a good idea to repeat the test on another day, reversing the temperature factors, to make sure it was temperature and not fatigue that made the difference. Generally, the brain works best at 68°F (20°C) and 40 percent humidity. However, what may be comfortable for others may not be comfortable for you.

Take Your Temperature

Our brains are affected by not only the environmental temperature but by our internal temperature, which rises and falls in a twenty-four-hour pattern. Your body temperature is probably highest in the late afternoon and lowest in the morning. Your brain will function best at certain times of the day that can be marked by how warm or cool your body is. Here is a chart to track your temperature, your cognition, and your mood at various times of the day.

Save four crossword puzzles from newspapers or buy a puzzle book. Take your temperature as soon as you wake up, mark it on the chart, note your mood, and then do as much of the puzzle as you can in ten minutes. Write down how much you finished—a quarter of it, a third, half, three quarters, or all.

Take your temperature and do a puzzle at noon, at 5 P.M., and at 9 P.M. Record your temperature, mood, and how much of the puzzle was completed. The rest of the day and evening, record just your temperature and mood at various times. Repeat the process for the next two days.

By looking at the chart, you should be able to see the body temperature and the time of day at which you function best. Keep this in mind and try to schedule your most challenging intellectual tasks at your peak time and your routine, automatic tasks at your low time.

Time	Day 1			Day 2			Day 3			
	Temp-erature	Mood	Puzzle	Temp-erature	Mood	Puzzle	Temp-erature	Mood	Puzzle	Average Temperature
7 A.M.										
8 A.M.										
9 A.M.										
10 A.M.										
11 A.M.										
12 P.M.										
1 P.M.										
2 P.M.										
3 P.M.										
4 P.M.										
5 P.M.										
6 P.M.										
7 P.M.										
8 P.M.										
9 P.M.										
10 P.M.										
11 P.M.										
12 A.M.										
1 A.M.										
2 A.M.										
3 A.M.										

Be Sensational and Feel Better

Your ability to sense your world inside and out is what makes you uniquely human and provides you with the pleasures of life. John Keats wrote to his friend in 1817, "O for a life of sensations rather than of thoughts." What the poet did not realize is that without sensations, there can be no thoughts, and without thoughts, there can be no sensations. Our ears, eyes, nose, mouth, and skin provide the information from the internal and external environment that is processed by our brains; and, in turn, our brains signal our organs about the meaning of what is being sensed.

By becoming more aware of the power of your senses, by performing the exercises in this chapter and the others in the book, you will help to increase and maintain the fitness of your brain.

3

Enhancing Coordination and Motor Skills

Remember a time when you dipped your foot into water that was either freezing cold or very hot, and in less than a second you bent your knee and withdrew your foot? Why didn't you fall over when you did that?

The nerves in your foot carried the message of the uncomfortable water temperature to your brain via your spinal cord. Then your brain sent a message down through your cord to flex your leg and withdraw your foot. Meanwhile, your other leg received the message to maintain extension and thus keep you from losing your balance. Such responses occur very rapidly and without your attention because they are built into your marvelous systems of nerve connections within your spinal cord. The cooperation of your brain, spinal cord, and muscles are more efficient than any machine ever invented by humans.

Pick up a cup.

Do you realize the tremendous cooperation required between your brain, nerves, and muscles to accomplish that feat? Your brain had to send signals to your shoulder, arm, wrist, and fingers. Your elbow had to bend. You had to reach out. Your fingers had to close and grasp, feel the weight of the cup, and then lift it up in the right direction—all in a series of rapid, precisely coordinated movements. Then your fingers and arm had to send back a message to your brain: "Mission accomplished!"

You picked up that cup without thinking about it, and yet just the ability of your thumb and fingers to make a pinching movement is one of the major reasons you are prime among the primates and all other creatures on earth. Of course, if you had to figure out how to pick up a cup every time you did it, you wouldn't be able to concentrate on anything else. A large part of movement, therefore, is both involuntary and outside your consciousness.

Dr. Ziaul Hasan, an associate professor of physiology and one of a number of researchers belonging to the Motor Control Group at the University of Arizona, gives another example. When you write with a pen on paper, you involve movement in your wrist and fingers. If you write on the blackboard with chalk, he says, the results are still very much the same, "But look at what you are doing. You are making entirely different movements using the shoulder and back. The muscular involvement is completely different and has nothing to do with what you did with pen and paper."[1]

It cannot be that you remembered a sequence of muscle contractions when writing on paper because that would not help you write on the board. How do you make that transition from one situation to another?

Investigators have discovered that your brain has prerecorded instructions, a "computer program," for virtually every movement. The natural computer program for your hand is stored in an area specifically set aside for it in your cerebral cortex. Just as a writer wouldn't use an accounting program as much as he or she would a word-processing one, the brain allots more space to some databases than to others. The more sensitive the surface of your body, the larger its "map" in the brain. Thus the amount of your brain tissue that contains input from your hands is quite a bit larger than that for your entire back and your legs. The space assigned to individual fingers varies greatly. It has no relationship to the size of your hand but has to do with the way you use your fingers.[2]

Scientists now believe that you can increase the area of the brain assigned to your fingers by increasing your use of them.[3] This was demonstrated in monkeys who were trained to maintain continuous contact with a disc for about fifteen seconds to obtain food. The disc was always available in the home cage and provided the only source of food. Moving the disc resulted in about two and a half hours of skin stimulation. The task required a high level of attentiveness. The experiment was conducted for several weeks. Detailed electrophysiological maps of the hand area in the brain were studied before stimulation was begun and several months after the repetitive hand use had ended. Significant alteration of brain areas resulted from the heavy, behaviorally-controlled hand use.

These studies reveal that brain maps for the fingers can be altered substantially in adult monkeys, a fact that contradicts the widely held notion, the researchers said, that area maps in the brain are strictly anatomically determined and are subject to modification for only a short while after birth. It also helps to explain the possible mechanisms underlying the acquisition of skill by practice, such as piano playing or sports.[4]

Animal studies also show that when a programmed area is dam-

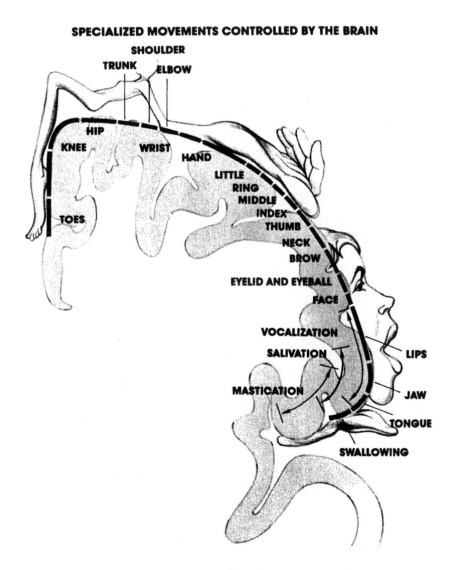

SPECIALIZED MOVEMENTS CONTROLLED BY THE BRAIN

aged or an inputting mechanism, such as a finger, is not working, the brain can compensate for it by expanding the area assigned to other input mechanisms, such as the other fingers.

For example, when researchers tested monkeys who had lost their fingers, the area in the cortex representing the lost digits were at first "silent" when electrical signals were recorded. However, over time, the silent zones became responsive to tactile stimulation of skin surfaces surrounding the amputated digits, leading the researchers to conclude that in an adult, "brain maps" can be altered by use. That is why to perform at a superior level, such as with the piano, you have to practice, practice, practice!

No one knows exactly how the new maps are drawn, but it is believed that fibers running from the motor area of the brain to the spinal cord are organized in such a way that each small motor brain map, controlling a particular movement, is surrounded by a "fringe" of motor nerve cells that have only a partial influence on that particular movement. When the main brain map becomes damaged, the fringe area may eventually take over. If such shifts could be enhanced, then certainly many accident and stroke victims would benefit and so would healthy people undergoing brain changes due to aging. Recent efforts on the behalf of people with paralyzed limbs is proving that it is possible. When a limb is paralyzed, there is an interruption in transmission between the control center, the brain, and the outlying stations, the limbs.

Although textbooks maintain that neurological deficits that persist more than six months are permanent, researchers at the University of Massachusetts have been proving that those "downed wires" can be bypassed or reconnected to reestablish transmission of nerve signals. Professor Walter P. Kroll and his colleagues at the university have been using Functional Electrical Stimulation (FES) and reestablishing movement years after function has been absent. Kroll, a professor of exercise science, said his most spectacular case was a thirty-three-year-old man whose left arm had been paralyzed since he was nine. After treatment, the man was able to gain independent control of his fingers and to flex his elbow enough to feed himself.

Kroll, who began his research nearly two decades ago with a grant from the U.S. Army, said his aim at the beginning was to gain a better understanding of how the brain controls movement. He and his other researchers have now concluded that the human brain has computer-like "programs" for various movements. By analyzing those muscle signals with a computer as the unaffected limb is moved, they can imitate the muscle pattern with electronics. The muscle pattern developed from the unaffected limb is then fed to the muscles of the immobile limb by electrical stimulation.

The amount of movement recovered after FES treatments depends upon a number of factors, including the length of time the limb has been affected, severity of the muscle and nerve damage, and the general health of the individual. However, Kroll and his colleagues feel that they are finally able to communicate directly with the brain in "a language the brain understands."[5]

We have also found at the New Jersey Neurological Institute that patients paralyzed for a number of years can be "taught" to move limbs again through electrical stimulation and biofeedback. Biofeedback is a technique designed to reduce tension by viewing or hearing responses in the body not normally felt. Electrodes or cuffs are attached to the body. When alerted by a graph, a sound, or a picture on a TV screen to a change in muscle tension, for example, the person makes an effort to somehow produce more of the change. This biofeedback enables a person to gain greater control over the body's responses such as blood pressure, heart beat, and respiration.

The PET scan and the brain mapper are instruments that turn brain wave tracings into graphic pictures, showing that you can exercise your brain through selective stimulation.

The illustration on the next page graphically illustrates the brain activity of a paralyzed young man thinking about moving his legs. He can see on the brain map screen the area his thought of leg movement is stimulating. He had electrodes attached to his legs that read signals from his muscles to a biofeedback screen. He could see on that screen how the thought in his brain stimulated the muscles in his legs. The muscles then moved and were recorded on the graph. His thoughts stimulating the area of his brain involved in movement actually helped him regain some use of his limbs.

Increased understanding of the brain is rapidly being accumulated by neuroscientists. Thus old beliefs, such as the one about a lost brain function being irretrievable after six months, are being modified. The cerebellum is subservient to the cerebral cortex, the "thinking brain," for the highest level of movement coordination.

French researchers recently showed with new neuroimagery techniques that the patterns of brain activation during mental rehearsal of

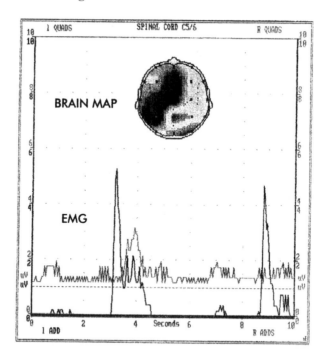

The above is a brain map of a young patient who is quadriplegic after spinal cord injury. This brain map (EEG) demonstrates the action of the legs commanded by patient's will to move them. *EMG* are electrodes attached to legs that respond to messages to move from his brain. The patient did move his legs here and could walk after biofeedback training. *(Courtesy New Jersey Neurological Institute)*

a motor act are similar to those produced by the act itself. The lead author of the French study, Angela Sirigu, and her colleagues pointed out in their report in the September 1996 issue of *Science*:

> Prediction is essential to many aspects of motor behavior, from postural compensation to the tracking of moving objects and the planning of complex trajectory. The capacity of the central nervous system to simulate and anticipate the behavior of the motor apparatus is a central issue not only in the experimental and computational studies of motor control but also in the study of mental processes. Humans can use this capacity to improve a motor skill or induce sensorimotor plasticity through mental rehearsal.[6]

Yogi Berra, the former Yankee catcher and much-quoted philosopher, put it this way: "Baseball is 90 percent mental and 50 percent physical."[7]

The coordination of the complicated signals that move your hands so that you can grasp a cup, pet a cat, or play the piano are processed by your *cerebellum*. The cerebellum is that part of the brain associated with coordination of muscles governing locomotion, posture, speech, and skilled movement. It lies at the back of your skull behind your brain stem and under the great hemispheres of your *cerebrum* and means simply, "lesser brain." It is much smaller than the cerebrum but looks like it. As in the cerebrum, the highest functions in the cerebellum are confined to the thin outer layer, which, like the cerebrum's, is folded and wrinkled to increase its area. The folds, in fact, are much deeper and more closely spaced than those of the cerebral cortex. If the cerebellum is split down the middle, the folds form a pattern that resembles a tree that medieval anatomists termed the "arbor vitae," or tree of life.

Why does practicing piano or tennis improve performance? It is believed to be because you are exercising your cerebellum. There is evidence that, as we learn to walk, speak, or play the piano, the necessary detailed control information is stored within the cerebellum where it can be called upon by commands from your cerebral cortex.[8] Cerebellar functions, such as coordination and balance can be modified. Younger people walk faster with good coordination. With age, this changes unless you maintain cerebellar activity.

Test Your Cerebellum

• With your hands at your side, close your eyes and touch your nose with one index finger and then with the other. Do this four times.

• Place a string on the floor or follow a straight line and walk heel to toe along it.

• Stand by a wall or chair so you can catch yourself, if necessary. Close your eyes and try to balance on one foot for the count of ten.

• Lie on your back with eyes shut and both legs straight. Then lift one leg and put its heel on the knee of the other leg. Try this test four times with each heel.

In a month, after you've done the cerebellar exercises we describe in this chapter, try these tests again. You may notice a difference in coordination.

❂ ❂ ❂

The cerebellum is being studied intensively today because it seems especially vulnerable to age. Elderly people generally require more time to prepare for and carry out a movement, pace themselves poorly in tasks requiring continuous performance, and fail to adjust their movements to compensate for errors. Why? In the past, such changes were thought to be related to decreased muscle strength or to the accumulation of fat with age. Now a National Institute on Aging–supported study of old animals suggests that changes in the brain may be responsible for many of the disturbances in movement that are seen in animals. Aged rats move their limbs less vigorously during prolonged exercise than do young adult rats. These movement disorders are strikingly similar to those seen in young adult rats with damaged dopamine-producing brain areas. There is evidence that the impaired function of aged rats can be reversed by administration of the amino acid L-dopa. It has long been known that dopamine-containing nerve cells of the brain play a critical role in movement, but recent research seems to indicate that dopamine may also affect the movement problems of healthy aged populations.[9]

Coordination is affected, including manual dexterity. Mark Williams, M.D., assistant professor of medicine at the University of Rochester, maintains that timing a person's manual dexterity is much more accurate than traditional tests for predicting his or her need for long-term care. Traditional tests include questions to assess an individual's alertness and tests to determine whether or not the person can perform the routine tasks of daily living.

Dr. Williams says that it must be determined why a person's speed of hand function is below a certain critical level. The loss of manual dexterity may be due to arthritis, a thyroid problem, or to medication, and may be improved with simple treatment. If, however, the loss is caused by a decline in the workings of the brain, then greater measures must be taken to increase the functioning of its motor centers or to make up for the deficit by other means.[10]

What can you do to enhance the function of your cerebellum?

Cerebellar stimulation—using coordinated movement—is one answer. Learning motor skills can, again, be compared to programming a computer. You can see a baby programming the cerebellum when you put a cup on his or her high-chair tray. The first time the baby tries to pick it up, the hands oscillate and knock the cup off. Presently, the cerebellum learns to judge how far to move the hand, how much to expand or contract the grasp.

In the adult, there is calculation of other fine measurements. For example, in tennis, the ball is hit toward you.

You instantly have to determine:

- How fast is it coming?
- Where should the racket be when it gets here?
- Do I need to move?
- What angle should I use?

When you become expert at tennis, your cerebellum plugs in the almost infinitely modifiable program for playing in a smoothly perfected manner.

You can be quite certain that Olympic athletes have cerebellums that operate with rapid communication between nerve cells and muscles. Because they constantly repeat their movements, their actions have become semiautomatic. If the cerebellum is damaged, however, through disease or injury, or infrequently challenged, one may be forced to consciously think through every fine movement, and those movements would not be as well executed as if they were done semiautomatically.

You may not become an Olympic athlete if the cerebellum with which you were born is not in top condition. But no matter what your age, you can improve what you have, often to a marked degree. Even if your competitor was born with a better cerebellum, motivation—that as yet unexplained phenomenon—can put you further ahead. It takes motivation and constant dedicated practice to improve.

One of the fundamental functions of the cerebellum is to help us learn and remember new movements, such as playing the piano. This suggests that the ability of the motor system to adapt to learning special movements may be significant in cases where damage to other parts of the brain requires reorganization. Under these circumstances the cerebellum may modify nerve function to compensate for impairment in the damaged parts of the brain.[11]

The cerebellum is vital to balance and movement, although the inner ear and other central nervous system components are also involved. The following exercises will help you improve balance and coordination.

Balance Exercises

The Old Book-on-Head Routine

Place a book on your head and walk forward along a straight line. You can place a string on the floor or follow a floor board or rug pattern, just as long as you follow a straight line, heel to toe, heel to toe.

Now, instead of walking forward along the line, walk sideways, stepping with your left foot and bringing your right to it. Then, when you reach the end of the line, go back, stepping with your right foot and bringing your left foot to it, still balancing the book on your head.

Repeat both heel-to-toe walking and side-stepping with the book on your head, but sing a song—any song—as you do it.

Backward Pickup

Place an object, such as a book or a can of food, on the floor. Walk twenty paces away. Make sure there are no objects to trip over and then walk backward without looking back while singing any song you choose. Bend to pick up the object at the place you believe it is.

Repeat this exercise three times, each time walking farther away and then back, but always singing something as you walk backward. This is to develop your sense of timing and hand-eye coordination.

Stork Balance

Do not do this exercise if you have difficulty with your balance or you have a condition that might be affected if you fall. As a safety precaution, stand near a wall or chair so that if you feel like falling, you can catch yourself.

Center yourself and consciously balance on both feet. Close your eyes and count to three.

Balance on your right foot, with your eyes still closed, to the count of three.

Balance on your left foot, with your eyes still closed, and count to three.

Open your eyes. Center yourself consciously on your two feet and count to five.

With your eyes open, balance on your right foot, with your left foot hooked behind your right knee, and count to three.

Center yourself on both feet and count to three.

Balance yourself on your right foot while holding your left foot in front of you in your hand and count to three.

Assume various kinds of body positions—use your imagination—while balancing on one foot. You might pretend to be the Statue of Liberty or an ostrich. Count to three.

Each day, try to increase the count while you balance with any of the above stances until you can get to fifteen while standing on one foot with your eyes closed.

Blanket Roll

Spread a blanket on the floor or on your bed and, with one hand over your head, roll to the right and then to the left. Roll right three times and left three times. Then roll yourself in the blanket with your head sticking out. This exercise helps you control your body while it is moving.

Table Topping

Lean over a table or desk with your feet on the floor and curl your fingers around the far edge of the table. Bend one knee and lift your bent leg toward the ceiling; do not allow your knee to turn out. Lift ten times. Repeat for the other leg.

Table topping will help to keep the communication going between your legs and your brain via your spine. Of course, don't do this if you have a physical condition that might cause you pain or injury while performing the exercise.

Shrug It Off

In a standing position, shrug your shoulders forward, up, down, and back. Your chest should elevate. Repeat ten times. This not only exercises control over your shoulders but helps relax tension that might interfere with performance.

Body-Movement Exercises for the Cerebellum

Line Dancing and Square Dancing

Excellent exercises. You are not only executing movement to music, you are following the directions of the caller. Any dancing, however, is good for your cerebellum.

Simon Sez

The children's game where you imitate the leader and try to avoid following directions when "Simon Sez" is not spoken is good for the same reasons that square dancing is beneficial: You have to pay attention, follow directions, and execute patterned moves.

Charades

In this game you try to describe a saying or an object to others by pantomime and body signals. Charades is excellent for your cerebellum, as well as the right side of your brain, because it employs body control as a substitute for speech.

Pat Yourself on the Head

Another child's game that can benefit your cerebellum is tapping the top of your head with one hand and rubbing your stomach with the other. Remember that? Do it for the count of twenty and then reverse your hands and repeat for the count of twenty. Do it as often as you can.

Handy Movements—Dexterity Exercises

The fine, coordinated movement of the fingers and hands depends a great deal on the cerebellum. By carefully following the exercises below, you can increase your dexterity.

Coin Stacker

Take one hundred pennies or dimes and stack them as high as you can. You might also try stacking coins of different denominations, but this requires precise placement.

Saucy Saucer

Take a saucer or ashtray. Dump some coins and/or buttons on the tabletop; then pick up and place as many of them in the dish as fast as you can—within thirty seconds.

Tweezer Pickup

Take a tweezer and several dozen loose straight pins. Put the pins on the table. Pick them up with the tweezer one at a time and place them in a saucer or ashtray. Place as many as you can within a count of thirty. Keep trying to better the number you can place in the dish each time you try the exercise.

Another Finger Exercise

Take eight straws (or eight pens or pencils) and pick up each straw with one hand until you have all eight in your palm. Then put down one straw at a time without dropping the ones remaining in your hand. Repeat the exercise with the other hand.

Hand-Eye Exercises

The extraordinary coordination between the hand and the eye involves fine movement. The following exercises will help strengthen the pathways.

Make the Connections

Connect the circles in order and as quickly as you can without lifting your pencil from the paper.

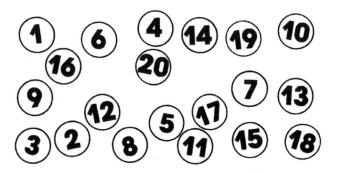

Connect the circles with a pencil line, but this time alternate between numbers and letters, keeping both in sequence.

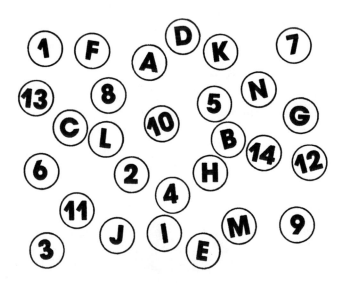

The Amazing Maze

Draw a path with your pencil from the opening in the upper right to the opening in the lower left without lifting the pencil from the paper and without crossing a line.

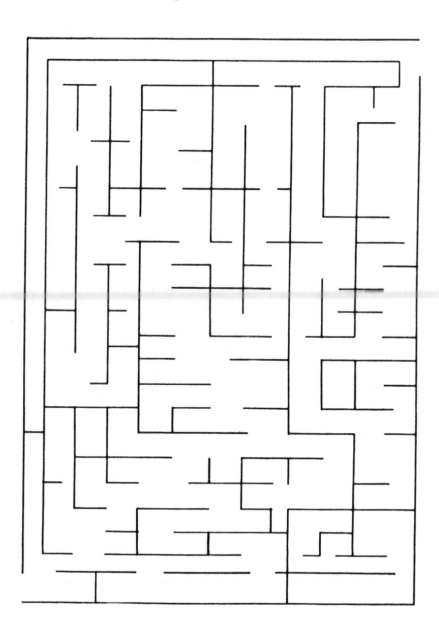

Cut It Out

Take a scissors and cut out figures or objects from magazines or newspapers. Try to follow the outline as closely as possible. If you have no scissors available or don't want to destroy the page, take a pencil and outline all the people or objects without lifting your pen or pencil from the page. Remember to stick as closely to the outline as possible, with all the little twists and turns.

Finger Fun

This is excellent for improving dexterity.
- Bend one finger at a time.
- Shake one finger at a time.
- Place your hands on a table and drum and tap your fingers.
- Sequentially move each finger in a half circle, starting from the little finger on your left hand.
- Hold your fingers together and extend and separate them one at a time.
- Spread the fingers of both hands and touch fingers to fingers in a clapping motion.

Put the Squeeze On

Take a box or a basket and put in a ball, a sponge, a soft cloth, and a piece of elastic (the kind sold in the variety store to repair undergarments). While you watch TV, without looking at the basket, squeeze and/or pull each item with one hand several times.

Play Jacks

The popular children's game where a ball is tossed in the air and a metal double cross is picked up before the ball bounces twice is one of the best exercises for your cerebellum. It requires hand speed and coordination. You start out by picking up the jacks one at a time, two at a time, and so forth up to ten at a time.

Bowling and baseball are two other recreational pursuits that are very good for your cerebellum. In bowling, you have to coordinate your movements and aim the ball at a distant pin. In baseball, you have to time your swing to hit the ball.

You know from experience that practice improves performance. Now prove it again by doing these brain builders for your cerebellum.

4

Brain Aerobics: Physical
Exercises That Go to Your Head

You have probably experienced that feeling of well-being after a brisk walk or a good game of tennis. Some joggers call it a "runner's high." Exercise has also been found to reduce anxiety and depression. Such mental effects have been attributed to the release of the brain's own opiates, *endorphins,* and to other nerve chemicals and hormones that are released with stimulating physical exercise.[1] Whatever the explanation, the fact remains that physical exercise can literally "go to your head." Some people actually become addicted to exercise.

There is controversy over exactly why and how physical exercise improves cognition, but there is general agreement that it can be highly beneficial. Cognition is the quality of *knowing.* It includes perceiving, recognizing, conceiving, judging, sensing, reasoning, and imagination.

As we get older, the reflex time required to prepare and carry out purposeful movement increases. The physiological response of reduced brain-wave frequency can be seen on the electroencephalograph. Slower electrical conduction along nerve pathways and slower reaction time also affects mental functions such as intellect, memory, attention, and perception.

In the recent past, declines in reaction times or voluntary movements were thought to be due to decreased muscle strength or accumulation of fat within the body. Now researchers believe that these changes are largely due to modification in the central nervous system. One of the theories is that some decline in function results from an insufficient supply of oxygen to the brain. It has been determined at the National Institute on Aging's Baltimore Gerontology Research Center that there is a drop in the amount of oxygen taken in by the lungs as we age. The circulating blood of a twenty-year-old man, the NIA studies show, will use, on the average, almost four liters of oxygen per minute. The circulating blood of a seventy-five-year-old will use only 1.5 liters per minute.

Reduced oxygen levels have been shown to cause a decline in the following neurotransmitter chemicals with which the brain's nerves communicate:

• *Dopamine.* A neurotransmitter present in high concentrations in the brain and proven in animal studies to be necessary for initiating fast movements and to be affected by vigorous exercise.[2]

• *Norepinephrine* (noradrenaline). A hormone from the adrenal gland (located just above the kidneys), it stimulates nerve cells, particularly those of smooth muscles, and constricts blood vessels.

• *Serotonin.* A blood-vessel constrictor present in high concentrations in the brain, it inhibits secretions in the digestive tract and stimulates smooth muscles. It also affects mood.

Each of these neurotransmitters has been correlated with human behavior, and the function of each declines with age.

Neurons that release these chemical messengers are in the base of the brain around the reticular formation, a structure highly involved in arousal and attention. Those nerves that secrete norepinephrine or serotonin reach to the hypothalamus, the limbic system, and other structures while the nerves producing dopamine project primarily to the basal ganglia. The basal ganglia, limbic system, and hypothalamus play a role in motor behaviors and emotional and motivational states. Sleep, pleasure, eating, reproductive behavior, and stress-related aggression all emanate from this area.

In one classic experiment, older rats housed in environments that provided for increased sensory and motor stimulation were shown to have an increased size and complexity of nerve networks. The area of transmission of the nerve chemicals—dopamine, norepinephrine, and serotonin—were larger than in rats in an ordinary environment. The researchers concluded that the changes may have occurred because of increased oxygenation of the brain tissues.[3]

It has been known for a long time that in patients with parkinsonism—which has been called the "stalking horse" of senescence—there is insufficient dopamine in the areas of the brain associated with movement. Hence, victims of parkinsonism have difficulty moving and may lose their balance in a manner we associate with the very, very old.

There is substantial evidence that movement, sensory stimulation, and even thinking results in an immediate increase of blood flow to the brain. The physical activities associated with an exercise program, in addition to improving the intake and use of oxygen and aerobic efficiency may, in humans, provide sufficient brain stimulation to promote physical changes in the brain and improve its function.[4]

Testing with human subjects seems to bear this out. Studies have shown that the reaction times of men who have maintained an active participation in physical activities such as racquet sports and running were significantly faster than those of age-matched sedentary men and little different from response times of much younger sedentary subjects.[5] Highly physically-fit older individuals scored higher on tests of fluid intelligence (the functioning of neurological structures) and memory retention than did less fit subjects.[6]

But did the better performance of physically fit older individuals reflect a predisposition for superiority in both athletic and cognitive abilities, or did their physical activity per se have the beneficial effect on their central nervous system functions?

If the latter were true, then could the central nervous system function of older people be significantly improved with a program of physical activity even though they have maintained a sedentary lifestyle for many years? Would aerobic exercises that emphasize increasing the oxygen in the muscles for strength and flexibility also help the brain?

There have been a number of studies to determine whether aerobic physical activity may really improve brain function.

In one study, sedentary individuals between fifty-five and seventy years of age were enlisted in a four-month aerobic-exercise conditioning program. They were compared to two age-matched control groups:

1. those trained with strength and flexibility exercises but not with exercises that increased oxygen intake
2. those not engaged in any supervised exercise program

The aerobically trained subjects, when tested, showed significantly greater improvement on neuropsychological tests and did better than either control group. The researchers concluded that the aerobic exercises promoted increased brain metabolism with a resultant improvement in neuropsychological test scores.[7]

In another study, researchers at Purdue University in Indiana enlisted seventy members of the faculty and business community between the ages of twenty-four and sixty-eight years to participate in a four-month physical fitness program.[8] The subjects were divided into the following groups:

High-fit young
High-fit old
Low-fit young
Low-fit old

Each group was given a ninety-minute exercise session once a week, beginning with warm-up calisthenics and then progressive running and self-selected recreational activities. Researchers found there was a marked improvement on fluid intelligence in all groups. Fluid intelligence, which is discussed in more detail in chapter 7, is the functioning of the neurological structures and is believed to decline with age unless some type of intervention takes place. The researchers found that regardless of age, the high-fit group had a significantly higher total fluid-intelligence score than the low-fit group.

The researchers said that oxygen, itself, may not play the major role in improved cerebral functioning, but it may affect the changes in brain chemistry that do.

The observed beneficial results of exercise—including its antidepressant effects—have been attributed to the release of endorphins, the neurotransmitters that cause feelings of euphoria, as mentioned earlier in this chapter. A study conducted by Dr. Daniel B. Carr, of Massachusetts General Hospital, and other researchers revealed that levels of beta-endorphin rose dramatically in the blood of nonathletes while exercising, and these levels increased even higher with regular training.[9] The beta-endorphins, in addition, augment tolerance to pain, which may also explain why some people run despite pulled muscles, chest discomfort, and other agonies. The morphinelike neurotransmitters are released by the brain and pituitary gland.

There is no doubt that there is a hormonal effect from vigorous exercise. For example, persistent and zealous exercise by female runners has been known to cause amenorrhea, an abnormal absence of or suppressed menstrual cycles. It makes sense then that fluctuations in the intensity of nerve communication caused by exercise can have a marked influence on the function of the nervous system. A popular hypothesis is that exercise improves the body's adaptation to emotional stress by increasing the efficiency of the adrenal glands, which release "fight or flight" chemicals such as norepinephrine in response to stress. You can see, therefore, how exercise that may affect the brain by increasing blood flow, oxygen, and metabolism could affect mood and cognition.[10]

There are those, however, who maintain that increased oxygen to the brain or changes in the neurochemistry of the brain, are not the cause of the improved mental functioning as reported in experiments such as the one performed by Dr. Carr. Some investigators think that the reason you "feel better" when you exercise is because you have enhanced feelings of self-worth and decreased psychological stress. Some investigators feel that the results are due to distraction from worry during exercise and that the social interaction and the feelings of mastery or accomplishment are the reasons people's mental functions seem to improve.[11] The actual result may be a combination of both theories.

In an effort to determine just how exercise does affect mood, researchers studied sixty-four subjects prior to and after either vigorous exercise or a hobby class. In general, the results support the claim that physical activity is associated with changes in mood and mental functioning. Although significant changes on several variables were also observed in the hobby group, the magnitude of changes from pre- to post-testing was greater for the exercise group.[12]

Among the parameters measured were anxiety, depression, self-confidence, adjustment, work efficiency, and sleep behavior. The hobby classes included painting, photography, typing, auto mechanics, and nutrition courses. The exercise class involved forty-five minutes of jogging and various other physical activities.

All took place between 6:30 P.M. and 7:30 P.M. to remove daily mood variations. The study showed that the exercise group felt more elated, less apprehensive, less serious, and less engaged in thought. They were less fatigued and less unhappy following exercises. Their scores on the profile of mood scale revealed that they also felt less anxious, less depressed, less angry, and less fatigued. The exercise class members had increased alertness and physical well-being.

The explanation as to why alertness is increased by exercise may be found in experiments in which ten men and eight women, age nineteen to twenty-four, were exercised to the point of exhaustion by researchers at New Mexico State University. After the volunteers had run on treadmills, their brain waves were recorded and they underwent tests of their perceptual and motor skills. The investigators found that there was significantly higher activity in the left hemisphere of the brain than in the right in the subjects and that this implied a more analytical mode of thinking due to the exercise.[13]

Exercises—particularly aerobic routines that increase the oxygen to your brain and stimulate the release of beneficial neurotransmitters—are good for your brain. The following exercises are aimed at doing just that. If you follow them faithfully, you should feel better and think better within three weeks.

Brain Breathing

We breathe twenty thousand times a day, but do we breathe well enough to supply our brains with sufficient oxygen? The single best indicator of fitness, according to many exercise physiologists, is how easily the body takes in and uses oxygen during work performed on a bicycle or a treadmill. The more physically fit, the better the oxygen metabolism.

If you don't believe your breathing can immediately affect your brain, take ten rapid deep breaths. It should make you feel light-headed because you have deliberately lowered the carbon dioxide in your blood.

The yogis have always emphasized proper breathing as a means of controlling body processes, including the brain and its by-product, emotions. How efficiently do you breathe?

Test Your Respiratory Efficiency

Lie down. Place your left hand on your lower abdomen and your right hand on your chest, just below your throat. Take several deep breaths as you would ordinarily, but try to exhale more deeply than usual. As you repeat this, you'll probably notice that when you exhale, your abdomen doesn't move much. Your chest is doing most of the work. This is called "paradoxical breathing" because it produces the opposite of what it should. Your respiratory system works against itself. Paradoxical breathing often follows breath holding that occurs when you try something new, are startled, or shift your attention. This is illustrated by the following:

1. Stand up quickly and then sit down again.
2. Snap your fingers about once a second. With each snap, shift your eyes so that with one snap you look to the extreme right and with the next snap you look to the extreme left. Repeat about ten to fifteen times.

What happened to your breath pattern? Didn't you hold your breath and then breathe shallowly with your chest? Such respiration is inefficient and tension-producing.

Belly breathing—using your abdominal muscles during inhalation —is a relaxed method of breathing and conserves energy.[14]

Try it. Start by sticking out your stomach and pushing it against your left hand. Then roll your breath up into your chest, pushing it against your right hand. Exhale even a bit more. Repeat this slowly, making your breathing rhythmic. Now, breathe into your left hand and then into your right, and then exhale very deeply. Do it to a slow count of eight.

The more you practice belly breathing, the more automatic it should become. You'll find yourself able to think and move better and even play sports better because belly breathing is an efficient way of taking in oxygen and getting rid of the waste product, carbon dioxide. And, when facing a stressful situation, if you increase and deepen your belly breathing, you'll send out the calming neurotransmitters, reducing the level of the excitatory ones from your brain.

Skull Shining

This is what yogis call this exercise because it brings a "radiant brightness" to your head. While sitting or standing, curl your lips over your teeth, leaving just a slit of your mouth open. Inhale deeply through your nose. Exhale forcefully through the slit between your lips in a series of short, distinct bursts of air. After completely exhaling, take several relaxed breaths and repeat once or twice more.

Breath Relaxer

This exercise will relax you and allow you to breathe more efficiently as it counteracts your "tightness" or stress. It is great to do while you are standing impatiently in line.

Stand with your knees slightly bent but not locked. Take a position with your feet about eight inches apart and bend your knees so that the weight of your body is in balance between the heels and the balls of your feet. The rest of your body should be in a straight line with your arms hanging loosely at your side. Let your belly hang out. Don't force it out but don't hold it in either. Belly breathe. Your back should be straight but not rigid, and your pelvis should be relaxed. Hold this position for two minutes.

Don't Forget to Yawn

The definition of a yawn is an involuntary opening of the mouth, usually accompanied by a deep respiration. It is often thought to be a sign of boredom. If you yawn, it indicates that you need more oxygen because you have probably been breathing shallowly. This commonly occurs when you are tired or under stress or have been sitting for a long time. Deliberately yawning and stretching at the same time is an excellent way of increasing oxygen to your brain.

Aerobic Exercises

Aerobic exercises are those that increase heart beat and oxygen intake. Active sports that involve running and jumping and bending will help bring oxygen to your brain. But many people cannot pursue team or formalized exercise. John Reeves, director of sports and recreation at the University of Rochester, describes the advantages and disadvantages of many common aerobic exercises, most of which you can do indoors:[15]

Jump Rope

This is a good and very inexpensive aerobic exercise. You can burn ten to twelve calories per minute at a fairly steady pace. You don't have to go outside and you can even do it in a hotel room. The disadvantage is that it is boring and, therefore, you probably wouldn't want to do it every day.

Racquet ball, Handball, and Squash

Each burns about eight calories a minute and is a good aerobic exercise. The advantage is that they are a lot of fun. The disadvantage is that special facilities and partners are needed to play these games.

Swimming

One of the best all-around exercises, it is especially good for cardiovascular fitness. It is very easily regulated to your capacity. It burns around eight calories a minute. The only disadvantage is that you have to find a place to swim.

Tennis

A fine form of aerobic exercise. It is a good competitive activity and very enjoyable, but again, you have to find a facility and a partner to play. It burns about six calories per minute.

Aerobic Dance or Exercise

Both burn from six to nine calories per minute. They are social activities and are good not only for the cardiovascular system but for flexibility. You may need a course with a leader and a group to spur you on. However, with programs on cable TV, on cassettes, and in books, it is possible to follow an aerobic dance or exercise program right in your own home.

Machines

Treadmills, rowing machines, and bicycles are fine methods of aerobic exercise. They burn about ten calories a minute. Such machines can be purchased starting at about $100.

Jogging will burn fourteen calories per minute and downhill skiing about ten calories per minute, but if you want to accomplish something practical while you exercise, consider doing any of the following as aerobic activity:

- scrubbing floors
- cleaning out the garage
- painting walls, outdoor furniture etc.
- washing and waxing the car
- gardening
- riding a bike or walking on errands instead of using the car

In addition to getting oxygen and blood to your brain with the above activities, you gain a sense of accomplishment and order. If the mundane aerobic activities don't appeal much to you, take a walk! A brisk walk, all agree, is one of the best and safest exercises. It will burn about six calories a minute and not cost you anything. You can enjoy the environment and appreciate life.

Physical fitness experts believe it is wise to do aerobic exercises two days a week to keep your cardiovascular system in good shape and to perform anaerobic exercises (strengthening without increased oxygen intake), such as lifting free weights, which should be done three times a week to keep muscles toned and strong. Before you start any aerobic exercise, first check with your physician and then do some stretching exercises. For example:

• Lie down with a pillow under your knees. Raise one arm slowly, then let it flop limply, trying to let it relax completely. Do the same with your other limbs in any order.

• Let your head roll slowly to the left, then to the right. Close your eyes. Let your jaw sag and inhale slowly. Close your mouth and exhale slowly, hissing or humming. Tense muscles—from toes up to neck—then relax them, concentrating on the difference between tension and relaxation.

• Draw up one knee slowly as far as possible. Then straighten it out and let it down easy. Repeat with the other knee.

• Sit in a chair and shrug your shoulders, then relax. Repeat three times.

• Stand and hold on to the back of a chair. Bend your right leg as if to kick your behind but do it slowly. Do the same with your left leg. Repeat three times.

• Reach for the sky with one arm and then with the other. Repeat three times.

• Hold on to the back of a chair and step back four steps. Bring your right foot forward and bend your right knee while you keep your left foot flat on the floor. Feel the stretch in your left leg. Hold for the count of three. Repeat the exercise, but this time bend your left knee and keep your right foot flat on the floor.

Get up, get out, and keep the "cobwebs" out of your head.

5

Fine-Tuning Your Brain with Music

We humans like music. We may not like the same combinations of notes and rhythms, but we use music to celebrate, attract, mourn, and move. Music is being studied intensively today, however, as a means of improving and maintaining brain and body functions. It has been shown to be beneficial for:

- muscular development
- physical coordination
- a sense of timing
- mental concentration
- memory skills
- visual and hearing development
- stress control

New investigations of the effects of music on brain function and the body have been energized by the reluctance of citizens to pay school taxes for so-called "nonessential" classes in music, and by health insurance companies who demand proof of music's therapeutic effects in treating illness.

Scientific studies have confirmed what we have known instinctively for ages—music has a soothing or stimulating influence on our behavior. The new information, however, demonstrates just how music impacts upon our nerves cells and brain function.

Michael H. Thaut, Ph.D., professor of music and biomedical engineering at Colorado State University, Fort Collins, and his colleagues first determined the effect of rhythm on normal subjects and found that people walked better to music then they did without.[1]

Then they experimented with ten stroke patients, half with the left side of the body paralyzed and half with the right. They were given rhythmic auditory stimulation thirty minutes a day for three weeks. At the end of this time, the patients had improved their walking—cadence, stride, and foot placement—compared with ten other stroke patients who had not been given auditory stimulation.

In addition to measuring patients' walking patterns, the Colorado group traced the electrical signal from their muscles used in walking to document the timing and magnitude of changes in the patients' gait.

The therapists also studied rhythmic auditory stimulation in patients with Parkinson's disease, and these patients, too, have obtained similar improvements in walking patterns compared with controls. They found that those with rhythmic auditory stimulation during a three-week, home-based gait-training program improved the speed of their gait by 25 percent and their stride length by 12 percent.[2]

"Two different pathologies—one hemispheric damage and the other damage to the brain stem basal ganglia—yet both respond to the same treatment," Dr. Thaut noted.

Thaut said that the metronome beat excites activity in the motor system of the brain, which helps organize and integrate complex movement. The primary clinical importance of music is not its emotional or motivational value, he said, but the neurological effects that improve motor control. When muscle activity is synchronized to auditory rhythm, it becomes more regular and efficient.

"The brain is organized in a complete pattern. Stride, length, step, cadence, symmetry, posture—everything, is centrally, not segmentally, related. So when one improves on one of these parameters, everything else comes into place. This fits in very well with modern theory about motor control," he explained.

Not only do patients walk better with auditory stimulation, but the effect lasts! The Colorado group has studied their patients after they have completed treatment and finds that they regain the walking pattern they acquired during rhythmic training. Patients can reliably reproduce their new walking pattern without further rhythmic cuing.

Exactly how does music work on your body? The sounds of music pass through your outer ear canal, strike your ear drum, and pass as vibrations through fluid to stimulate your auditory nerves, which then carry the message to your thalamus, your brain's relay station for sensory information. The thalamus, in turn, sends the musical stimuli to the area of your brain concerned with hearing. The auditory part of your brain then processes the music so that you recognize the song you've heard and its message stirs your memories or associations. This is a conscious process. But the music also has an unconscious effect. Mediated by your thalamus, the elements of music—pitch, rhythm, and intensity—directly affect your autonomic nervous system, which regulates breathing, heart action, motor function, and digestion. It also affects your hormones.

If you still doubt that music directly affects your brain, consider the dramatic cases of patients with musicogenic epilepsy. Their brains are overexcited by certain varieties of music, which cause them to have seizures. The gamut of stimuli is wide ranging, from serene violin music to jazz. In one case, a woman was affected by organ music. She tried to leave church before the instrument was played, but sometimes she did not make it out the door.

Music, if used properly, is a readily available, highly effective tool that you can use to improve both your brain function and physical abilities.

The ancient Greeks knew that. They worshipped Apollo, god of healing and music, and believed each musical mode, rhythm, and instrument created its own special response. Modern medical practitioners have only recently found out that the Greeks were right. In fact, there are now music therapists who use their skills to aid the disabled.

More and more therapists, however, are now aiding healthy people to improve brain function with music since there is increasing evidence that if you learn a musical instrument in adulthood, take up singing or really concentrate on what an orchestra is playing (there is a difference between hearing and really listening), these activities will help you:

- strengthen your body,
- organize your thinking,
- improve your coordination.

The cerebellum is devoted to the regulation of the sort of movements we execute when playing musical instruments. Current research suggests that one of its fundamental functions may be to help us learn and remember new movements, such as playing the piano.[3] Further, it is suggested that the ability of the motor system to adapt to learning special movements may be significant in cases where damage to other parts of the brain requires reorganization. It makes sense, therefore, that exercising the cerebellum with music may modify nerve function in the healthy and compensate for impairment due to wear and tear as the years pass.

Frank Wilson, M.D., chief of neurology at Kaiser-Permanente Medical Center, Walnut Creek, California, and an assistant clinical professor of neurology at the University of California, San Francisco, points out that it takes more of the brain to control the small muscles of the body that we use when we play a musical instrument than to control the large muscles we use when we swing a tennis racket.[4]

Dr. Wilson himself began music lessons at the age of forty. "At first, I felt clumsy, but then an amazing transformation seemed to take place. By the end of my sixth month, my hands were suddenly making music that I had been hearing in my head since the beginning."

He said he first became fascinated with how the human brain and body coordinate to produce music while watching his eleven-year-old daughter play Chopin's Fantasy Impromptu on the piano.

"It struck me that there was something wonderful going on. Learning to play the piano involves a wide range of human skills that we use in almost all our daily activities. I thought as a neurologist I should know about this process. I wanted to know how the brain functions when a musician plays a fast passage on a musical instrument. We all have the ability to do it, but, of course, we are not all willing to make the effort to practice until we can do it."

What about talent?

"First of all, talent is not very well defined, and in some sense, it is a destructive word. People use 'talent' to talk themselves or others out of playing an instrument. The key to success in music, as in sports, is having the right goals. If you set out to sound like a professional or try for the stage, your attitude is self-defeating."

He notes that if you consider yourself as a beginning music student the same way you would consider yourself learning a new sport, you will succeed: "Musical performance demands the same type of training needed by athletes. The only difference from a physical point of view between musicians and athletes is that musicians are concerned with the smaller muscles of the body—especially those of the hands and perhaps the mouth, and they rely on their hearing more than their vision."

He compares playing an instrument to jogging:

> Jogging has become popular because people aren't concerned with coming in first in a race as a measure of their suc-

cess. They are compelled by the knowledge that they are extending themselves and enjoying the experience. If they run a mile or more than they did the last time, or run the same distance faster than before, they have succeeded. The same can be true of music. If the musicians are compelled by the knowledge they are reaching new limits and sharing the experience with others—if in a band or group lessons—they are more likely to succeed. If you play a difficult piece more smoothly than before or move on to something even more challenging, that should be your reward. You do feel wonderful when you have mastered something that's difficult. It gives you a terrific lift.

The "lift" you get from music, Dr. Wilson and other researchers agree, is as much physiological as it is psychological. Did you ever consider why stereo is preferred over monaural music? According to researchers, it is because it stimulates more nerves in your brain. According to Dr. Manfred R. Schroeder, a physicist associated with AT&T Bell Laboratories in New Jersey, the more stimulation of the nerves, the greater the enjoyment.[5] He said nerve signals reaching the brain from the ears can work at cross purposes. If the signals are similar enough and if they arrive at nearly the same time, stimulation of the brain's nerves can actually be inhibited. Such may be the case with monaural music, which presents an almost identical sound in both ears. Since stereo, on the other hand, delivers different sounds to each ear, the auditory nerves send different messages to the brain. As a result, more brain and nerves are excited.

It is the pulsing or flowing of the music in time, and not the melody, that compels us to move.

Tempo, on the other hand, refers to the rate at which a piece of music is played. If rhythm makes us want to move, tempo affects how fast. It can pace our work and make it more fun. Just consider the popularity of jogging with earphones and of aerobic dancing.

How Music Affects the Brain

Music is a universal language in human culture, and yet the brain mechanisms involved in understanding music are still quite mysterious. With the use of high-tech instruments, neuroscientists are attempting to see how the human brain processes music.

A team of neurologists, Gottfried Schlaug and Helmuth Steinmetz of Düsseldorf's Henrich Heine University, took pictures of the brains of thirty classically trained musicians with perfect pitch who had the ability to identify any musical note without comparison to a reference note (a talent held by Mozart, among other famous composers and musicians).

In the study, the German researchers took MRIs (magnetic resonance imaging, computerized images) of the brains of thirty musicians and thirty nonmusicians. All the musicians in the study were the same age and all had years of classical training. All the subjects were right-handed, and Dr. Schlaug said that he had expected that the pictures would show a slightly enlarged structure on the left side, a pattern that is common for right-handed people. Instead, he found that in eleven musicians with perfect pitch, only the left temporal lobe was enlarged. It was about 40 percent bigger than their right temporal lobes. There was a slight left-side enlargement among musicians without perfect pitch, but not much different than the lobes of thirty *nonmusicians* in the study.[6]

Brain experts found this important because it is the first study to specifically and systematically relate a structure of the brain to an artistic talent.

"There is evidence that those with perfect pitch were exposed to music before the age of seven," said Schlaug, who is now at Boston's Beth Israel Hospital. "If you get exposed to music after the age of ten, the likelihood of developing perfect pitch is extremely low.

"We know from other of our studies that there are people who are extremely left asymmetric [have enlarged left temporal lobes] but who are not musicians and have never been exposed to music," Schlaug said. "This suggests strongly that it takes both 'nature and nurture' to create musical genius."

Schlaug says the team's interest in the temporal lobe was reinforced by a 1950s study of a German musician who suffered melody-deafness after a stroke, apparently as a result of damage to his temporal lobe.

Schlaug doesn't know whether the asymmetry and associated musical talent are inborn traits or whether they can be acquired through training,

"Pitch is a part of grammar," Dr. M. J. Tramo of the Department of Psychology, University of Montreal, Quebec, Canada, explains. "When you ask a question, the pitch rises. When you string individual speech sounds and sequences into sentences to express ideas, you begin to use pitch."[7]

He and his colleagues tested two patients with lesions on both sides of the brain in temporal regions behind the "temples." The perception of speech and environmental sounds were preserved: yet, the perception of music was impaired. As the processing of melodic but not rhythmic variations in musical sequences was selectively disturbed, the deficit cannot be attributed to a general impairment in auditory memory. These findings suggest that melody processing is not mediated by a general purpose auditory architecture but by specialized brain systems.[8]

Pitch is also an integral part of music. When the brain listens to music, Dr. Tramo said, it uses many of the same pitch detectors that are used in decoding spoken language.

Language involves the ability to hear words and to use them skillfully to express concepts fluently.

Music concerns the ability to hear and produce rhythms, melodies, and harmonies.

Some scientists think that language and music are two sides of the same intellectual coin. Cellular circuits that recognize language and music are found on both sides of the brain, said Dr. Jashed Bharucha, a psychologist at Dartmouth College, Hanover, New Hampshire, but the left side also contains regions that specialize exclusively in language and the right has some regions that exclusively serve musical perception. In the brains of musical idiot savants—individuals who are severely mentally retarded but who are talented in music—the dichotomy is especially pronounced.[9]

This is also evident in stutterers and some stroke patients. Country music singer Mel Tillis is a stutterer. However, he is able to sing without stuttering. Stroke patients who cannot speak may be able to sing.

Dr. Robert Zatorre, a psychologist at the Montreal Neurological Institute and Hospital, points out that music can be imagined because we have stored representations of songs, melodies, and the sounds of instruments. These representations can be stimulated internally, he said. When a song is "imagined," the cells and networks that are activated are identical to those used when a person actually hears music coming from the external world. But when songs are imagined, Dr. Zatorre said, parts of the visual cortex also light up, suggesting that tonal patterns evoke visual imagery patterns.[10]

"We don't know what triggers musical imagery," Dr. Zatorre concludes, "but it is very common for people to wake up in the morning with songs running through their heads."

Brain mapping shows that musical networks also extend into the brain's emotional circuits in the limbic system. People report strong emotional sensations when they listen to music, saying for example, that they feel like their hair is standing on end or they have "a lump in their throats."

Some Psychological Effects of Music

Baby Brains and Music

The effect of music is evidently an inborn phenomenon. A number of experiments have shown that music stimulates movement in both newborn and unborn babies. Elaine Nichols, unit coordinator of Monmouth Medical Center, Long Branch, New Jersey, reported that Bach, Beethoven, and Brahms are used in the hospital's nursery to stimulate the brains of unborn and newborn infants. Vivaldi is also played because its violins and high and low extremes of pitch are better heard by babies. She recommends that fathers sing to their unborn children because the father's deeper bass tones are better received through the amniotic fluid than the mother's higher tones.

In several centers in the United States and Israel, unborn babies are being stimulated by the application of headphones from portable cassette players to their mother's abdomen. Fetal breathing movements and body movements are now considered as a good index of an unborn child's well-being. The influence of fetal well-being was examined in twenty women to whom pop and classical music was played via earphones. An ultrasound scanner allowed direct observation of the fetus's body movements and breathing movements. The researchers found a significant decrease in breathing activity in fetuses while their mothers listened to their preferred type of music—whether it was rock or Beethoven made no difference. When music that the mother liked came through the headphones, it soothed the unborn infant.[11]

The Effects of Rhythm and Tempo

Humans have long used music to make repetitive tasks easier, such as "toting that barge" and "lifting that bale." Rhythm and tempo make these movements easier. Researchers at Stanford University, Stanford, California, set out to determine just how brain, muscle, and music work together to achieve greater ease of movement.

Monica Grenicr Safranek, Gail Koshland, and Gay Raymond at Stanford University first studied the electrical patterns emanated by flexion and extension of the elbow in women eighteen to thirty-five years of age while performing a motor task without listening to rhythm. The subjects were asked to hit three targets in the following pattern: Target I, one time; Target 2, three times; Target 3, two times. Each woman, the Stanford researchers reported, had their own personal rhythm. They practiced the target hitting until they became skilled at it. The Stanford investigators point out that one assumption made about a skilled motor performance is that it reflects the most efficient recruitment of motor units (nerves and muscles that work together) because these units are activated more quickly and in greater synchronization than during unskilled performance.[12]

When an even rhythm was played, the electrical signals recorded from the elbow muscles were decreased and created a more even pattern. When an uneven rhythm was played, the signals from the elbow muscles increased and were irregular, in a pattern similar to when a person is unskilled at a motor task.

The researchers concluded that an even rhythm aids efficiency in movement and produces action similar to that usually seen in skilled performance of motor tasks.

Rhythm and tempo are not only useful in coordinating muscle action, they are also a means for altering mood. We use music and voice for biofeedback training at the New Jersey Neurological Institute. For some the use of fast rhythm and marching tempo have a negative effect. One subject asked that the music be changed to a more classical type because "my daughter plays that fast, loud, music and it bothers me!"

Music and Emotion

A certified music therapist with a great interest in music therapy for the healthy, Shelly Katsch, M.A., C.M.T., of New York City, former vice president of the National Association of Music Therapy, points out that music does very much involve the right side of the brain, where emotions and feelings are located.[13]

Music communicates emotions—the very deep level of feeling that you sometimes can't express in words. Furthermore, playing an instrument or working with music directly affects your sense of creativity and accomplishment. You can develop a stronger sense of self—of self esteem. You can reexperience the joy of sound making. Many adults have lost the natural love for making sounds that children have because as youngsters they were told to "be quiet" when they made noise by vocalizing repetitive sounds. They became inhibited."[14]

She and other musicologists say that when you hear the sounds that you produce with your voice or a musical instrument, you can relearn how to make joyful sounds.

Emotionally arousing experiences are often called "thrilling." A *thrill* is a subtle nervous tremor caused by intense emotion or excitement (such as a pleasure or a fear), producing a slight shudder or tingling through the body.

Dr. Avram Goldstein of Stanford University used music to bring thrills under some kind of experimental control. To test the hypothesis that thrills, like other emotional responses, may be mediated in some manner by endorphins—our self-produced brain opiates—Dr. Goldstein carried out an experiment attempting to block them with naloxone, a medication that blocks the effects of opiates.[15]

Volunteers listened to music of their choice through earphones. If they experienced a localized thrill of the lowest intensity, Dr. Goldstein reported, they raised one finger. If the thrill was more intense, they raised two fingers, and if it was very intense and spread to distant parts of the body, three fingers were raised. The duration of the thrill was indicated by the length of time the fingers were raised.

The subjects were tested before and after intravenous injections of naloxone.

Males and females reported similar results. By far the most frequent site of origin of thrills was the area of the upper spine and the back of the neck. Spreading occurred typically in a radiating or sweeping pattern, upward over the scalp and outward over the shoulders and arms and down the spine.

The naloxone lessened the "thrill" and Dr. Goldstein surmised this was because it blocked the brain's own opiates.

Any kind of experience that arouses emotions can elicit thrills in those who are susceptible. The common element appears to be a confrontation with something of extraordinary beauty or of profound and moving significance. Our own "right kind" of music is also very effective.

The thrill, Dr. Goldstein said, is an emotional response involving the autonomic nervous system probably mediated by endorphins.

Music and Pain

William Congreve wrote in 1697, "Music has charms to soothe a savage breast, to soften rocks, or bend a knotted oak." In the 1840s, Florence Nightingale, the founder of modern nursing, noticed that injured British soldiers who listened to music healed faster and experienced less stress. Now modern researchers are studying the cellular basis for such a result.

In research conducted by Dr. Beverly Whipple of the Newark campus of Rutgers, the State University of New Jersey, she says listening to music measurably increases pain thresholds.

"When you have another stimulus, such as music, coming into the brain, it serves as a gate that blocks the interpretation of the pain," explains Whipple, associate professor at the College of Nursing. "While other research has theorized about the gating mechanism of listening to music, this project demonstrates that there is a quantitative increase in pain thresholds brought about by music listening."[16]

If you are in pain, would it better to listen to soothing or stimulating music to encourage your brain to pour out its own opiates?

Some researchers have found that stimulating, rather than relaxing, music has the most broad-ranging effect on pain. Others maintain that hard rock or jazz stimulate nerve endings and thus make us more alert to pain.

In the study, subjects listened to music to determine how much pressure they could withstand on their fingers and how much heat they could tolerate before asking to have the tests terminated because they were uncomfortable.

The volunteers then were asked to listen to soothing music for fifteen minutes, after which measurements were taken. Following a resting period, they then were asked to listen to fifteen minutes of stimulating music, and again pain and tactile thresholds were measured.

When the subjects listened to soothing music, they experienced an elevation in pain detection and pain tolerance threshold levels, and were able to withstand greater levels of pain. Stimulating music, however, elevated both pain thresholds and tactile thresholds, indicating that such music not only may help to reduce the pain, but also may act as a distractor.

"The great things about these findings is that anybody can do it," said Whipple. "Anybody can turn on some music and may gain relief from their pain. This gives people an added measure of control over their bodies and what happens to them. They can become the ones who are in control, so the pain no longer controls them."

Clive E. Robbins, Ph.D., director of the Nordoff-Robbins Music Therapy Center at New York University, one of the pioneers of modern music therapy, points out: "Some say the brain is fundamentally programmed so that the organic connections are symphonic rather than mechanistic."[17]

Music and Intellect

In addition to the emotional lift music making can give us, music can also help improve our ability to think.

Researchers at the University of California, Irvine, have been studying music training as a possible "exercise" for higher brain function.

"If we can establish a relationship between early music training and abstract reasoning skills, it would have enormous consequences, particularly for children from disadvantaged backgrounds," according to Frances Rauscher, Gerard Research Fellow at the Center for Neurobiology of Learning and Memory.

Using standardized tests of abstract reasoning, Rauscher has measured the mental performance of three-year-olds as they begin music training.

By examining individual scores on the different puzzles and games, Raucher is trying to determine which skills are most enhanced by musical training.

Gordon Shaw, UCI professor of physics, who works with Rauscher, says: "Consider music as a sort of prelanguage, that, at an early age, excites these inherent brain patterns and enhances their use in other higher cognitive functions. Because this internal neural language should be the same for various higher brain functions, we predict that music training at an early age is 'exercise' for higher cognitive function."[18]

Recent work at other institutions, such as the University of Arizona, showed that infants as young as five months understood simple addition and subtraction. If there is a link between inherent brain structures that give rise to music and other higher abilities, the UCI researchers suggest that music can strike a chord in these structures, acting as both a window to examine higher brain function and as a stimulating exercise to accelerate development.

We learn to recognize patterns in our music, just as we recognize patterns in our language. The music "speaks" to us in pitch and rhythm.

Researchers at Stanford found that babies as young as six months old showed a preference for what is called an appropriate musical phrase.

The babies could control how long each excerpt played by looking at a light or a checkerboard in the test booth. When they looked away, the music stopped.

"These findings are interesting for two reasons," said Anne Fernald, associate professor of psychology and an expert on infant language development. "First they show that infants appreciate musical phrase structure in musical forms they have never heard before. And second, it seems that hearing a 'well structured' piece of music first helps the infant appreciate differences between well-structured and poorly structured pieces."[19]

Researchers at the Music School in Providence, Rhode Island, wanted to investigate the connection between music and math. Research has shown that music students often perform at a higher level than other students in standardized tests.

The study team, made up of scientists and musicians, decided to test students with standardized math tests before and after they were given musical instruction.

The two-year study focused on ninety-six first- and second-graders divided into eight classes. Four of the classes were dubbed "test arts" classes and exposed, for an hour a week, to a method of musical training called the *Kodaly method* and a visual arts class emphasizing drawing methods that progressed from simple to complex. The Kodaly method was developed by a Hungarian composer more than sixty years ago to train students in basic musical skills. It also teaches the reading and writing of music. It stresses the development of an inner musical ear through unaccompanied singing and features games, dancing to folk music and hand signaling. It employs the senses and movement to stimulate the brain with music and the children have fun doing it.°

The remaining four classes received standard variety music and art classes—students learned songs while a teacher played a piano and constructed various craft projects. After seven months, the schools administered standardized tests and compared the scores with those from a year before.

None of the designers of the study were prepared for the results. Those students in the enriched program showed a meteoric rise in math skills—from 38 percent of the class performing at "grade level," where they were supposed to be in skill, to 77 percent. The control group, which started out with 47 percent at grade level, moved to 55 percent. In addition, those children who showed below-average reading skills caught up to average if they had been in the enriched arts program. Some of these children were from inner city, disadvantaged families and they not only caught up but forged ahead of their classmates.

Martin Gardiner, Ph.D., a biophysicist and research director of the Music School, concluded there were two results: "Learning they can master such challenging skills could foster a change in the students' general attitude toward learning and school. Also, learning art skills forces mental 'stretching' of the variety needed in math."

The questions that are most intriguing: Does music actually do something to the brain cells of children and can it do something similar to those of adults?

Mozart Improves Marks

College students who listened to ten minutes of Mozart before taking a standard test of spatial intelligence raised their scores by a significant margin, according to a study conducted by the University of California, Irvine.[20]

Reporting in *Nature*, Dr. Frances Raucher, the lead researcher, described the study of thirty-six college students. The students were given the three tasks to test their spatial reasoning following three listening conditions: Mozart's Sonata for Two Pianos in D Major, a relaxation tape, silence. The students' average spatial IQ score after listening to

°For more information, contact: Glenys Wignes, Executive Director, The Organization of American Kodaly Educators, 1457 S. 23rd St., Fargo, ND 58103-3708; phone: (701) 235-0366.

Mozart was 119 compared to 111 after the relaxation tape and 110 following silence.

What About Studying to Music?

Some persons have found that listening to soft music while studying may aid retention, especially when you hear the music again. The association may help recall. This may work with trying to memorize a small amount of material, but, generally, music playing during intensive study is distracting. Trying to listen to music and learn at the same time doesn't work for most students. As you read in the information about pain above, there is a "gate" theory, and trying to force several stimuli at once through the doorway to the brain may cause a block.

Take a Mini-Music Vacation

Since music exercises your brain cells and affects the area of emotions, you can give your brain and body a mini-vacation by stopping what you are doing, relaxing in a chair or on a bed, and playing the music of your choice. Soft, sweet music, of course, will probably be more relaxing to you, but if you like country or rock and roll, that may help take your mind off reality for the moment and release some of those endorphins from your brain.

Music Workouts for Your Brain

Donald Shelter, Ed.D., professor of music education at the University of Rochester's Eastman School of Music, New York, explains why music can be intellectually stimulating:

> There is a difference between hearing and really listening to music. The listener is intellectually involved. When you really listen, you go beyond just appreciating the surface things. You identify, discriminate, classify, synthesize, detect formal and stylistic features in music. You make a conscious effort. When you perform, you are doing all those mind expanding things the listener does, but you also add the physical functioning as well. You move your fingers and hands. Your muscles, joints, bones have to receive and exercise your commands. It is mental and physical skill. It demands concentration. There is an esthetic satisfaction and feedback that is self-renewing. Whether you just listen

to or perform music, that feedback involves accomplishment, challenge, and self-fulfillment. It is a peak experience.[21]

Think of a Song

Think of a song you know very well. Try reciting the words silently to yourself, without the melody in mind, and stop when you first stumble. Now, try it with the melody—you should get further.

Dr. Jon Eisenson, a Stanford professor emeritus of hearing and speech science, uses music to treat patients unable to speak because of strokes or other brain injuries that affect the left side of the brain. Music and melody fall under the right hemisphere's jurisdiction, and Eisenson maintains that even the most severely impaired speechless (aphasic) person's recovery can be enhanced if the significant role of the brain's right hemisphere is recognized.[22]

As pointed out before, singing and speaking come from a different area of the brain.

So singing is good for your brain. It makes words easier to remember and offers more efficient feedback than speaking. Alone, it stimulates a different area of the brain than speech and it provides an emotional release.

What if you can't carry a tune?

David Sudnow, a former sociology professor at New York University who left university life to teach piano to adults, maintains that anyone can carry a tune.

"If you think you can't carry a tune, it was because someone inhibited you as a child and now you can't open your mouth and let the sound out." He maintains he can teach anyone to carry a tune in a few sessions.[23]

According to Karl U. Smith, a retired University of Wisconsin psychology professor, you need only look in the mirror to see if you have real musical talent. He maintains that *left-faced* people are better singers. He studied *facedness* for many years and says that Frank Sinatra, opera singers, and famous composers all are *left-faced*.

You can tell your facedness, Smith maintains, by looking in the mirror and seeing which eyebrow is higher, which eye is more open and which side your smile is more pronounced. Muscular control of the face, he explains is divided. The right side controls the consonant-forming lips and tongue, while the left side steers the vowel-shaping cheeks and throat. Stronger vowel makers make better singers, he continues. His theory is that you can't develop acute perception of tone without being able to produce tones to some degree.[24]

So you're right-faced and can't be a great singer, but can you play the piano?

The professor-turned-music teacher David Sudnow has been very successful in New York City using electronic piano keyboards and video tapes to teach adults to play music "by ear" in four to eight weeks. He says that your hands can learn to play a musical instrument much as your feet can learn to dance. It becomes automatic.

He compares improvised music making—playing by ear without notes—to ordinary talking. In the former, there is an instrument lying outside the body while in the latter, all of the parts being used are body parts. Yet, a true incorporation does occur and it makes sense to speak of the instrument as a genuine extension of the body, just as it makes sense to say that the blind man comes to feel the pavement or the wall through the tip of his cane.

Many physical effects can be derived from using your body to make music. In fact, listening to music has been found to lower blood pressure and affect galvanic skin resistance and respiratory rates. It has been shown to affect the pattern of electrical activity of the muscles and nerves, and thus its physiological effects on function have been measured.[25]

What other physical fitness benefits can you achieve with a musical instrument?

Rochester's Dr. Shelter points out that playing woodwinds improves breath control and increases oxygen to the brain. (However, check with your physician if you suffer from high blood pressure before taking up a woodwind.)

"Singing is one of the best therapeutic measures for both mind and body," Dr. Shelter maintains. "It gives you the opportunity to extend vocal sounds. Ordinary speech does not extend sound but a long note does. Thus, singing exercises the larynx and vocal cords and feeds back to the area of the brain that receives music and voice sounds. Exercising any muscle strengthens it and, of course, the breathing apparatus is made of muscle. Further, singing is fun, particularly if you sing familiar songs and tape them on a recorder. You can enjoy listening to yourself."[26]

He says the piano and violin are excellent for finger manipulation and can improve hand-eye coordination.

Music can eliminate loneliness and solitude, which can interfere with cognition. It is the only art in which you can be both the doer and the audience. You can perform just for yourself and not be dependent upon others for feedback.

How much will you have to practice to benefit the physiology of your brain?

Neurologist Frank Wilson, M.D., says that most of the physical and intellectual benefits of music are derived from practicing. He practices an hour before he leaves for the office each day. Most experts suggest an hour a day. Some say you can break it up into fifteen-minute segments. Others say it takes at least fifteen minutes to warm up and fifteen minutes to begin to derive benefits from the practice. In any event, Dr. Wilson recommends patience because it will take six months to a year before you really reap the full benefits of learning to play an instrument in adulthood.[27]

Choosing a Teacher

You can learn by yourself but a good teacher can help you progress. Make sure the instructor's personality meshes with yours. Many are used to teaching children and not adults. The old European conservatory type of teaching with lots of scales and exercises is passé; playing songs right from the beginning is the preferred method today. It's more enjoyable. Good sources of information about teachers are friends who are already taking lessons, local music stores, school music instructors, and Ys and other community centers. Group instruction is widely available and allows you to share your experience and make new friends.

Selecting an Instrument

The piano, most experts agree, is probably easiest for an adult because you don't have to learn to make a tone on it as you do with wind instruments or violins. Piano keyboards have become computerized and portable, just like guitars, so you can carry them around. There are many second-hand instruments around, so before you lay out a great deal of money, borrow one or buy a second-hand one to see if you really wish to continue with your lessons.

The following is an evaluation of the degree of difficulty for various instruments provided by the American Music Conference, the national group composed of instrument producers and others interested in promoting the playing of musical instruments.

• **Easiest:** Autoharp, electric keyboard, bongo drums, recorder, chord organ, ukulele, and conga drums
• **Fairly easy:** Accordion, drum set, acoustic guitar, electric guitar, banjo, harmonica, concertina, and mandolin
• **Average:** Alto saxophone, flute, tenor sax, baritone sax, organ, trombone, clarinet, piano (upright), tuba, cornet/trumpet, sousaphone, xylophone
• **Fairly difficult:** Bass viol, cello, French horn, viola, violin
• **Most difficult:** Bassoon, harp, English horn, and oboe

6

How to Improve Your Memory

When you forget what it was you came into a room to get or where you put something, are you afraid you are developing Alzheimer's?

If you are a student, do you find that you know your material well before an exam but the minute you sit down to write the answers you go blank.

There is a lot more to memory than just remembering.

Are you as intelligent as you once were?

Would you like to be more intelligent than you have ever been?

Intelligence is the capacity to learn.

Learning is based on the acquisition of new knowledge about the environment.

Memory is its retention.

Research psychologists and neurobiologists have just recently been able to actually see the changes that occur in the chemistry and electrical output of the brain cells as learning takes place and memories are stored. What had been only surmised in the past can now be proven. By learning new things and by using your intellectual capabilities more efficiently, you can actually change the physical properties of your brain. And these changes can take place no matter what your age!

As we have noted before, people do not use the full capacity of their brains. Some use more than others. There are geniuses among us and "sloths." We all use our brains better on some days than others. You know, for example, that when you are harassed and tired, you may not be able to remember your own phone number or where you put your car keys. The information is stored in your memory but you can't recall it. Your learning ability may not be impaired, but your ability to perform is temporarily reduced.

We discussed in earlier chapters how information is fed into your brain through your senses. If you need glasses and don't wear them, your brain is not going to be able to perceive written directions and learn a new way to put something together. If the environment is so noisy you can't hear your lover say "I love you," you won't be able to recall that tender moment. Your sense perceptions have to be keen and your state of alertness, emotions, motivations, and environmental situation all have to be conducive to learning and retention if beneficial changes in your brain cells are to occur. The acquiring of new and the recalling of past information are necessary for "working out" the brain and for prime thinking.

Neurobiologists are using powerful microscopes to *see* and minute electrodes to *hear* those changes in a single brain cell as learning takes place.

They can see that when a cat learns or when its brain is stimulated electrically, its brain forms new connections between neurons by the branching out of their dendrites, the spiderlike "sensors" emanating from the shaft of a nerve. Similar nerve growth has been observed in hamsters and rats. These results are interpreted to mean that nerve cells show changes in their form and function as they take part in increased "internal traffic."

Marian Diamond, Ph.D., and James Connor, Ph.D., of the Department of Physiology and Anatomy at the University of California at Berkeley, reported in 1980 that they were able, for the first time, to show that there can be an actual increase in the dendrites in the cortex of the aged brain.[1]

Changes have also been measured in the synapses—the gaps between nerve cells where information is exchanged and the nerve cell is either fired into action or blocked from reacting. The learning results not only in adding or subtracting synapses, but by altering the strength of such contacts.

There is much that is still unknown about how we remember. It has long been noted that the hippocampus is involved in the storage of memory. When the hippocampus is removed for medical reasons, patients can still retrieve memories stored up to the point of that removal. We can see with the PET scan and brain scan that when someone remembers something, several areas of the brain "light up."

There is also what is sometimes called "flash bulb" memory. It involves the release of stress hormones. Where were you, for example, when President Kennedy was shot? If you were old enough to understand the news of the event, you undoubtedly remember what you were doing. That is "flash bulb" memory imprinted indelibly in your brain.

Stress hormones can also interfere with memory. In an interesting experiment performed at Washington University, St. Louis, Missouri, investigators enrolled nineteen normal adults. They gave some stress hormones on four consecutive days or an inactive placebo for four consecutive days. Blood sampling and cognitive testing were performed prior to the start of treatment, during treatment, and again one week after treatment stopped.[2]

The participants were given a standard audiotape presentation of a paragraph with about twenty-five bits of information. At the end of the reading, they were asked to repeat exactly what they had heard. After thirty minutes, they were again asked to repeat the information.

In subjects who received inactive placebo, paragraph recall improved at each testing, consistent with the idea that practice improves performance. In those who received the stress hormone, however, there was a significant decrease in memory performance after four days of treatment. Memory, as measured in the cognitive tests, did not return to normal one week after treatment concluded.

John Newcomer, M.D., the principal investigator, notes: "I think it is important that we didn't find significant impairment in memory performance until this treatment condition had been underway for four days ... If we had to extrapolate to a 'real world' situation, we wouldn't expect to see this kind of change in memory performance after just one day of physiologic stress. However, there could be such an effect after prolonged periods of high stress."

He says no one in the study noticed any cognitive changes or any impairment in day-to-day functioning, but the researchers could measure the difference.

It is also important to note, Dr. Newcomer says, that the impairment was reversible: "I think it speaks to the flexibility of this system and the reversibility of these kinds of changes in the brain."

Sudden stress can imprint a memory and constant stress, after a while, will impair memory function. Even a little stress without much emotional involvement can interfere with recall and learning. This is often evident in older people and students who know the answers to questions but under the stress of the exam, they have difficulty with re-call.

Without memory there can, of course, be no learning or high intelligence. But how do the changes in brain cells produce a memory? How and where are memories stored?

Try to go back as far as you can in your memory. Whatever it was you remembered was in your head for almost as many years as you've been alive. You have just used your long-term memory.

Now, pick up a phone book and select any number. Close the book and write it down. Wait one minute and, without looking at the number again, try to write it down. Did you forget? The phone number probably remained with you just long enough for you to write it down the first time. In this case, you have used your short-term memory.

Your short-term memory can hold between five and ten pieces of information. Unless you repeat to yourself what you are trying to remember, the data is typically forgotten in less than a minute. Your temporary storage system is used, for example, when you recall what someone said a moment ago. This small-capacity "working memory" does play a critical role in your reasoning and comprehension.

In contrast, the capacity of your long-term memory is vast. It normally contains records of enormous numbers of facts and experiences. You can preserve information for many years without making any conscious effort at all to retain it.

In the mid-70s, researchers at Bell Laboratories in Murray Hill, New Jersey, studied both short-term and long-term memory.

To test short-term, Max Mathews, Sc.D., David Meyer, Ph.D., now of the University of Michigan, and Saul Sternberg, Ph.D., gave subjects a set of numbers to learn and then asked them if certain digits were in that list. They measured the time it took a person to answer.

Based on the speed with which the group in general replied, the Bell researchers concluded that our minds can search through a memorized list at least three times faster than our eyes can. We are capable of making a mental search at the rate of twenty-five to thirty digits per second.

Long-term memory, the Bell researchers believe, is arranged like a thesaurus: words with related meanings seem to be stored "near" each other in the brain. Nearness, however, may correspond to either physical proximity or richness of nerve connections. They base their belief on the fact that we can recognize and pronounce a printed word faster when it is related in meaning to an immediately preceding word—such as *doctor* to *nurse*—rather than if it is unrelated—such as *doctor* and *vase*.

One logical explanation of why long-term memory is probably stored this way, they said, is that retrieving a word from long-term memory temporarily increases nerve activity in the locations of other nearby words. This "overflow" activation reduces the process needed to recognize a related word, and thus speeds up reaction time.[3]

Now you can see why "association," a technique used in mnemonics is so effective.

Speed is essential when using long-term memory. The search rate of thirty items per second estimated for short-term memory would be much too slow for finding a particular word among the thousands stored in the archives of your brain's long-term memory. Reading, writing, or speaking a single sentence would take several minutes if we had to rely on this recall time. The speed of searching our long-term memory is measured in milliseconds. We can, for example, recognize the meaning of more than 100,000 words in less than a second.

But how does short-term memory become long-term?

No one knows for certain, but there are clues. It is well known that a person who suffers a concussion can't remember what happened immediately before the accident, so-called *retrograde amnesia*. A patient receiving electroshock for depression also suffers from memory problems. The jolting of the brain in both cases somehow short circuits the processing of short-term memory into long-term.

We must be able to file what we experience for future use or we can't function in the world. One of the greatest quests today in psychology and neuroscience is to find how and where memory is stored in the brain.

It is known that the storage of data in our brains requires three basic things:

1. *REGISTRATION.* Our brain must receive the information from our senses.
2. *CONSOLIDATION.* The information has to be stored either short-term or long-term.
3. *RETRIEVAL.* We have to be able to call up that information when we want it.

The first major breakthrough in the scientific understanding of memory occurred in 1936 when Canadian neurosurgeon Wilder Penfield, M.D., touched an electric needle to the surface of the brain of a patient who was awake, and that patient began recalling an event as vividly as if it were happening right then and there. Dr. Penfield's experiment has been repeated by others, but no one has yet identified the exact location in the brain of the memory bank or banks.[4]

There are hints based on work with people whose memories have been affected by injury or disease. It has been determined, for example, that damage to a portion of the side of the brain, the medial temporal cortex, does not interfere greatly with a person's ability to learn, but that person forgets whatever he has learned almost immediately. He can't change short-term memory into long-term. Damage to another part of the bottom of the brain, the diencephalon, which contains the control centers for the endocrine glands and the basic drives, limits the ability to form new memories but leaves almost intact the ability to retain what was previously learned. In certain cases of tumors and intractable epilepsy, half the brain may be removed and yet the memories stored and the ability to record new ones may remain intact.

Today, research on memory is primarily physiological. Scientists now believe that memories are stored electro-chemically. This belief is based on the second big breakthrough in the study of memory, which occurred in the 1970s. That's when neurotransmitters—the chemicals secreted by the brain's nerve cells that carry messages between nerve cells—were discovered. They hold the key to the acquisition, consolidation, and retrieval of memories.

Since our long-term memory is stored quite efficiently, what we want to improve is our short-term memory and our retrieval of long-term memory. These are the problems about which many people begin to complain after the age of thirty-five years. In fact, it is so common that researchers call it "benign senile forgetfulness."

We all have experienced meeting someone and being unable to remember that person's name. *Nominal memory,* which seems to give many people over thirty some difficulty at times, involves being able to recall what someone or something is called.

We all have also experienced forgetting where we put something, such as our glasses or a paper. While "losing" something can happen at any age, it does become a more common phenomenon in those over thirty. *Spatial memory* involves knowing where an object belongs, including ourselves. When was the last time you stood before the refrigerator or a filing cabinet and said, "Now, why did I come here?"

You may suddenly recall a person's name or remember where you put your keys or why you entered a room. Why did you have difficulty remembering? How were you able to eventually recall the name or the place you were seeking?

Psychologists have long been aware that emotions play a significant role in the memory process. Sigmund Freud found that during therapy patients were able to recall incidents that had long been forgotten. He reasoned that certain events had been forgotten because they were upsetting to the patient. He called this process of "motivated forgetting" *repression.*

A similar process occurs in amnesia. After undergoing a particularly traumatic event, such as a criminal assault, the subject may have no memory of the entire episode, or some of the details may be lost to him. According to current theory, sometimes amnesia occurs when people are unable to face the reality of their own behavior or the situation in which they find themselves.

An interesting phenomenon of memory retrieval is illustrated in the film *City Lights.* Charlie Chaplin saves a drunken millionaire from suicide and becomes his friend. The millionaire, when sober, forgets who Charlie is and has him thrown out. Drunk again, the millionaire embraces Charlie as his friend. Scientific experiments have confirmed this phenomenon. Subjects given alcohol and made drunk were asked to hide a set of keys. Unable to retrieve the keys when sober, they were made drunk again and could easily locate the lost objects.

Exactly how we remember and why we forget is still not clear to scientists, although it is known that physical and emotional factors affect our memories. Depressed people frequently complain of poor memory—especially short-term memory. Older people, as well, sometimes find it difficult to recall current experiences but can remember events that took place fifty years ago. Despite the fact that there is much yet to be learned about memory, you can increase your ability to turn short-term memories into long-term. It takes motivation and practice.

Memory training can produce spectacular results. In a report in *Science,* for example, researchers at Carnegie-Mellon University, Pittsburgh, described how an undergraduate student with an average memory and average intelligence engaged in memory training for about one hour a day, three to five days a week, for more than a year and a half. He was able to increase the amount of information his short-term memory held from seven to seventy-nine digits. Furthermore, his ability to remember digits after the session—his long-term memory—also improved. In the beginning he could recall virtually nothing after an hour's session; after twenty months of practice, he could recall more than 80 percent.[5]

The system used at Carnegie-Mellon was actually first reported in 477 B.C. and is widely used to improve the memories of stroke victims. It is called mnemonics—the principle of associating unknown material with something familiar: The advantage is that it relieves the burden on short-term memory because recall can be achieved through a single association with an already existing item stored in long-term memory.

The trick is to make the association between what we want to remember and what we have already remembered vivid.

Association Practice

Associations are the links that hold the intellect together. The following is an exercise that will help you make associations. Try to find the word that fits with each of the other for words. For example, what word would you attach to:

SET BURN LIGHT BEAM _____

If you associated "sun" with them, you'd have had the answer. But it is the practice of associating the counts, not the right answers. When you have spare time waiting for an appointment or are sitting at a boring meeting, try to make up your own lists. Here are ten more examples.

1. LESS DEAD UP REAR _____
2. WAY TIDE BACK WHITE _____
3. ORDER MAN BOX AIR _____
4. LIGHT TO ONE SOME _____
5. LIGHT STOUT GOOD BIG _____
6. WEATHER STOCK CARD NEWS _____
7. EXAMINE WORD DOUBLE ROAD _____
8. HAT CHAIR LIGHT FLYING _____
9. AT SKI ROPE HIGH _____
10. LACE TIE BREAK LINE _____

Answers: 1. end; 2. water; 3. mail; 4. day; 5. hearted; 6. report; 7. cross; 8. high; 9. jump; 10. neck.

The following are two further tests of your memory. You can judge for yourself how much you need to improve it.

An Exercise for Retrieval and Speed

With a kitchen timer or your watch, write down as many five-letter words as you can in two minutes. You can practice this exercise whenever you want with six-, seven-, or eight-letter words.

List Memorization

Look at the following list of words for five seconds. On a blank piece of paper write as many as you can remember.

DOG	WINTER
CAT	STONE
BIRD	WHITE
SHOVEL	WILL
SKILL	WENT
HOUSE	TEN
ROBIN	BOOK
GRANT	LIFE
HORSE	LATE
CRAG	STAR
ELIZABETH TAYLOR	HONOR

How many did you write down? Probably no more than ten, but undoubtedly you remembered Elizabeth Taylor. If you established associations as readily with the other words, you would have had a perfect score.

Face Identification

Look at the pictures on page 99 and the first names under them for twelve seconds. Then turn the page, look at the pictures again, and try to write down the first names on a piece of paper. Again, if you had practiced association—"hooking" what is to be remembered with something already filed—you would have gotten a perfect score.

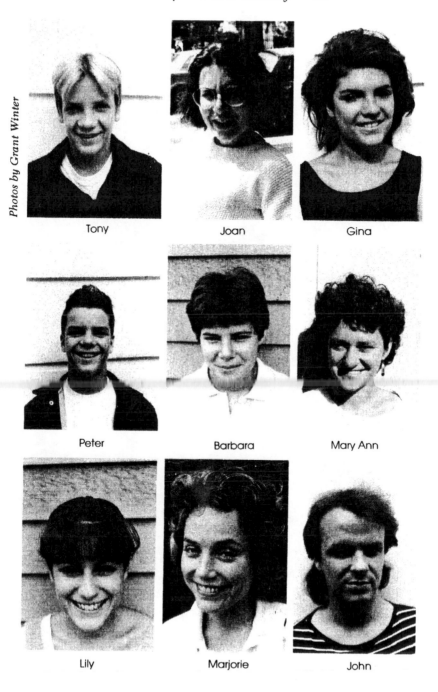

Tony   Joan   Gina

Peter   Barbara   Mary Ann

Lily   Marjorie   John

Photos by Grant Winter

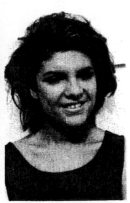
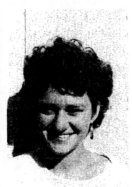
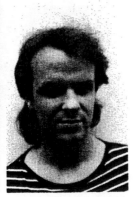
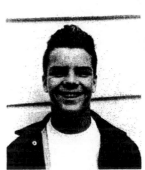
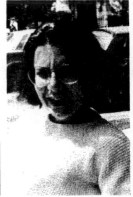
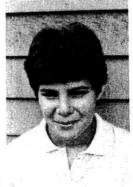
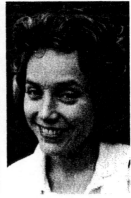
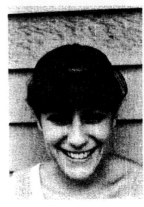

Further Memorization Exercises

> If, in my retirement to the humble station of a private citizen, I am accompanied with the esteem and approbation of my fellow citizens, trophies obtained by the blood-stained steel or the tattered flags of the tented field, will never be envied. The care of human life and happiness, and not their destruction, is the first and only legitimate object of good government.
>
> —Thomas Jefferson, March 31, 1809

- Write a headline that describes the meaning of the paragraph.
- Underline the important words first.
- Sing the words in the entire paragraph.
- Read them aloud.
- Now close the book and write down as much of the paragraph as you can remember.

How did you do?

More Retrieval Exercises

Select a book you have not read. It can be a novel or nonfiction. After each chapter, write a summary of it. After you have finished reading the entire book, write a summary of the book without looking at the chapter summaries.

If it is a novel, on paper, retrace the events in the main character's life, starting at the book's conclusion and then going backward to the beginning. If it is a nonfiction book, start with the main conclusion of the book and retrace the steps the author took to arrive at that outcome. Then look at your chapter summaries to evaluate how well you consolidated and retrieved the information.

Now memorize the following:

> *Some weigh their pleasure by their lust,*
> *Their wisdom by their rage of will:*
> *Their treasure is their only trust;*
> *A cloaked craft their store of skill.*
> *But all the pleasure that I find*
> *Is to maintain a quiet mind.*
>
> *My wealth is health and perfect ease;*
> *My conscience clear by chief defense;*
> *I neither seek by bribes to please,*
> *Nor by deceit to breed offense.*

Thus do I live; thus will I die;
Would all did so as well as I!

—Sir Edward Dyer,
from "My Mind to Me a Kingdom"

Which was easier? Singing lines, underlining, and rhyming all help you remember because they form "connections." Poetry and music exercise the right side of your brain.

The more concrete the item to be recalled, the more unusual or ridiculous the image created to associate it with, the easier it will be to remember.

Suppose you want to remember a shopping list of bread, eggs, flour, and orange juice. The first thing to do is to picture a loaf of bread breaking open and an egg falling out. Then picture a pitcher of orange juice being poured into the hole in the flour bag. Each item is linked to the subsequent one via the ridiculous image. By using mnemonics, stroke patients who couldn't remember the days and the months before, were soon able to master the whole list of U. S. presidents.

Another ancient trick is to think of a room and picture putting each thing you want to remember on some object in the room. Suppose you wish to remember to pick up the clothes at the cleaners, take a letter to the post office, and stop for some bread. Picture your living room. Picture clothes on the arm chair, a letter on the coffee table, and bread on the sofa. The same would work for a long number. Suppose you wished to remember 143054. You could picture 14 on the chair, 30 on the coffee table, and 54 on the sofa. Then you can easily remember the number 143054 when you picture walking into that room.

Practice Visualization

Since, as pointed out above, creating a mental image aids memory, you want to practice this skill. You can do so, for example, by doing jigsaw puzzles or even better yet, by making your own. Take any picture from a magazine and cut it in large pieces. Make the cuts curved and angled. Mix up the pieces and then put them together again. This also helps hand-eye coordination.

Another visualization exercise can also be done very simply. You don't have to be an artist. Take a piece of paper and, without looking up from the paper, sketch the furniture in the room. You can do this whenever you are bored during a meeting, while waiting in an office, or just for fun. Sketch a room that you remember from your childhood home or a school room. Putting what you visualize in your mind on paper is a good brain exercise.

What Else Can You Do?

Stay in Good Health

People with poor circulation, collagen disease, or other physical problems suffer more of a mental decline than those who are in reasonably good health. Successful treatment of physical ailments may improve memory.

Check Your Diet and Medications

A number of drugs in common use, such as those for ulcers, anxiety, or high blood pressure, may affect one's ability to remember. A diet that is not sufficiently nutritious (see chapter 9) can also affect the ability to remember. If you suspect either your medications or your diet, check with your physician. Sometimes merely a change in medication or prescribed dietary supplements may improve memory significantly.

Pay Attention

One of the problems identified with people who have difficulty learning is that it is often not their memory at fault, so much as their concentration. There is a decline in the ability to discriminate and retain after fifteen to forty-five minutes of studying at any age. Therefore, you should take five- to ten-minute breaks. An intermission gives the brain a chance to *consolidate* and *organize* what has just been run through it.

Say It Out Loud

When trying to remember something—especially short-term—say it aloud. Hearing something helps you retain it. Noise can interfere with your retaining something short-term, so try to keep your environment quiet while you are learning something new.

Use Categories

You can name all of the states in the union more easily, for example, if you do it by geographical divisions rather than randomly. Remember researchers believe related memories may be stored next to one another. Grocery lists can be remembered more easily, for example, by product categories, such as "dairy," "meats," "canned goods."

Use Cadence

If you set what you are trying to remember to music or make it into a rhyme, you will remember it more easily.

Break Things into Chunks

The nine-digit zip code proposed by the postal service was two numbers too long for most people's short-term memory. Therefore, if you have to remember a long number, break it into chunks. A number such as 555619101 can more easily be remembered as 55   619   101.

Review

When you review, according to current research, you strengthen the connections and associations between the nerve cells in your brain, but it does little good to repeat and repeat what you are trying to memorize in rapid succession. Since initial consolidation of information from short-term to long-term is thought to occur within ten minutes of the event, the first review should take place ten minutes after you've completed your study. Further reviews should be done one day, one week, and one month, and then six months after the study to make maximum use of consolidation.

Memorize Something Each Day

The more you use your brain to retain information, the more you will be able to do it efficiently. The more you remember, the more you can remember. Take your dictionary and a pad and pencil. Learn one new word a day. Write it down in the pad. The next day, learn another new word and write it down. Review the one from the day before as well. Keep doing that each day and you will not only increase your vocabulary, you will be exercising your memorization ability.

Intend to Remember

Psychiatrist William James wrote in mid-century: "What we are interested in is what sticks in our consciousness. Everything else we get rid of as quickly as possible."

Always Repeat Instructions

When given instructions or directions, repeat aloud what has been said or written. This will help clarify the steps in your mind and you will be able to remember them better. One of the theories about why this works well is that the right half of the brain is used for visual memory and the left half for verbal memory. By looking at instructions and then repeating aloud, the whole brain is employed to remember.

Organize, Organize, Organize

This is one of the most important memory aids. Many middle-aged and older people who made an effort to put things in proper order when younger become careless once they find there are less demands upon their time. Before beginning the day or a project, think through the sequence you will follow. Do things in order of priority, naturally, but if you have a task that is tedious, try to do that first. You'll be less likely to forget projects that are more interesting.

Remember Names

One often-tried method of remembering a person's name when introduced is to make a picture association with the name. Mrs. White could be associated with a white duck, for example. Repeating the name after someone gives it to you helps as does asking the person the origin of the name, if that is appropriate. You can also rhyme the name in your mind. "Jones" with "bones," for example. Anything that works to "fix" the person's name in your memory. Use all your senses. *See* the person and remember the features. *Touch* the person with a handshake or a pat on the shoulder. *Hear* the person's voice—tone and cadence. If that person is wearing a perfume or an after-shave lotion, you can even use your sense of *smell.* (although in our society, it is not polite to sniff. It is in some other cultures, however: In some Arab societies, it is considered proper etiquette to inhale another's breath.)

Use Your Common Senses

Some of us remember what we have seen better than what we have heard. And others remember what they have heard better than what they have seen. Which one are you? Remember the house where you grew up? Can you picture it clearly—the furniture, the yard, the kitchen? Can you remember the discussions at the dinner table or hear your mother giving you advice as you left for school? If you can picture the house better than you can remember the sounds there, you are more visual than verbal. What about your smell memory? Actually, many scientists maintain that it is everyone's best memory. Once you have identified a smell, you never forget it. In any case, it is through our senses that we gather information. We can use all of them to help us remember. When you are trying to memorize something, be conscious of how it smells, sounds, or looks. Try this experiment to prove how "sensing" can help you remember. Take a bottle of toilet water or a bar of sweet-smelling soap. Sniff it and read a paragraph and note the meaning of the paragraph. Sniff the perfumed object again. Tomorrow, take the perfume object and sniff it again. You should recall the paragraph immediately.

Put Away Your Calculator

A good exercise for the left side of your brain is to add, multiply, and subtract without the aid of a calculator. If you don't keep refreshing your memory with the answers to mathematical manipulations, you will have increasing difficulty retrieving the answers to numerical problems. To help yourself keep the machinery oiled, count up to sixty by threes, starting with the number two. Count back from one hundred by sixes. Whenever you are waiting in line or you can't sleep, try your own version of this number exercise.

Since math is one of the skills that fades rapidly in adulthood, especially with the use of a calculator as a crutch, here are some easy math exercises to refresh that part of your brain that handles numbers. *Do not use a calculator!*

- Tom walks a half mile in ten minutes. How far will he have gone in an hour?
- Jane, a store owner, has a business loan of $3,000 due in twenty days. She has $1,800 toward the loan. How much will she have to earn each day to be able to pay off the loan?

- Mary was five feet, four inches tall. She was shocked when the scale told her she weighed 174 pounds. On a fourteen-week diet, she lost three pounds each week. How much did she weigh at the end of the regimen?
- Henry was collecting money for a charity. His wife gave him $10; his boss gave him $45; his friends Pete, Ralph, and Sam each gave him $32; and he added $50 himself. How much did Henry collect?
- A party was held at a club. The club has a total of 2,644 members. 1,824 showed up for the event. About what percentage of the members did not come?

Other Memory Helpers

You have done everything above to give your brain a workout, but in your busy life distractions are many and you forget where you put something or that you had an appointment. The following are some tried-and-true reminder techniques:

Make a Note

Carry a small notepad or one of those tiny recording devices—they are now even available on a key chain—and record what you need to do in the near future, including finding your car in a mall shopping center. New cars often have *"car finders."*—you press a button and your car blinks its lights or sounds its horn for you. You can also put a piece of tape on your hand and write yourself a reminder. If necessary, you can use those small self-stick papers to write reminders on the telephone, refrigerator, brief case, car, or anywhere you deem necessary. You can also call yourself and leave reminders on your home answering device.

Charge Your Mind

When you hide something or place a letter to be mailed, concentrate on the act of placement. You may even repeat out loud: "I am putting this package here to be mailed later." You can also put your keys or glasses in the same place all the time. Always have copies of crucial keys and keep a set in your wallet; give an extra set to a relative or to your neighbor.

Answers: 1. 3 miles; 2. $60; 3. 132 pounds; 4. $201; 5. about 31 percent.

By the Numbers

More and more computerized facilities in our lives need PIN numbers, including banks and bank cards. Why not have the same PIN for all of them? The last four digits of your social security number or a loved one's birthday may be easy to remember. If you still have trouble, you can plant a fictitious name—such as your favorite character from a book or a movie star—in your address book and put your pin number by the name.

Use a Kitchen Timer

Association, as we pointed out, is a powerful memory tool. If you have to remember to call someone or return to a task after answering the phone, turn on your kitchen timer for an appropriate span, and when it rings it will remind you of what you were supposed to do.

Make an Exit List

If you are the kind that worries that you forgot to turn off the lights or the oven or leave food for the dog, make a list that you can paste on your usual exit from your home. Scan the list before you leave and put your mind at ease.

Scientists may still have a lot to learn about your memory, but one thing is certain—you have to exercise it! The purpose of this book is to help you gain self-mastery. If you really want to, you can "refresh your memory."

7

Expand Your Capacity to Learn

Francis Crick, who won the Nobel Prize for his work with DNA, the genetic imprint of a cell, has said that a single nerve cell is a dumb thing. What is astonishing in his view is that the powers of the human mind emerge in their entirety from these dumb units.[1] How did Crick use the nerve cells in his head to revolutionize the field of genetics? How did Einstein use his neurons to come up with the theory of relativity?

Einstein did not talk until he was three years old. He did poorly in school and may have been dyslexic, yet he overcame the disadvantages he had to revolutionize the world of physics.[2] Scientists studied Einstein's brain but could not determine if it was much different than the brains of ordinary people.

Learning is more than having a high IQ or being great at memorizing. It basically involves two endeavors:

1. accumulating and storing information efficiently in your brain, as described in the previous chapter
2. knowing how to use that information when it is needed

Your chronological age is really no excuse if your intellectual performance is not up to par.

The idea that great regressive changes in intellect can be expected as part of the normal aging process is not valid. Some people not only show no deficit as the years go by, but they actually increase in intellect.

Psychologists in the 1930s said that intelligence peaks in the late teens. In the 1940s they said intelligence peaks at age twenty-five. In the 1950s, psychologists said the peak was in the thirties, and now psychologists are telling us that one type of intelligence peaks in the forties while another peaks between the ages of sixty and seventy.

How can age and intelligence be accurately evaluated in humans? There are two basic techniques:

1. *Cross-sectional.* You take a group of people in different age groups—the twenties, forties, and fifties, for example, and compare how they do on tests.
2. *Longitudinal.* You begin studying people in their teens and test them periodically as they age.

The classic study was conducted by K. Warner Schaie, now of Penn State University and formerly director of the Gerontology Research Institute at the University of Southern California in Los Angeles. He completed a twenty-one-year study of intellectual performance in aging adults. During the course of the study, Schaie and his colleagues examined several thousand healthy volunteers living in the community and ranging in age from twenty-two to eighty-one years. Subjects were called back at seven-year intervals for retesting. The most positive and provocative finding of this work is that at all ages the majority of people studied maintained their levels of intellectual competence—or actually improved—as they grew older. Even between the ages of seventy-four and eighty-one, almost 10 percent of the people tested performed better than they had at younger ages.[3]

There are basic problems with both cross-sectional and longitudinal studies. Max Fogel, Ph.D., supervising psychologist of Mensa, the organization of people who score in the 98th percentile on IQ tests, explains why: "First of all, young people today have a better education. Then there is the motivational factor. Younger people are more eager to do well on tests. They are more interested in impressing others, and they are more socially active."[4] On the other hand, he explains, the longitudinal studies are done over a period of years. The selection factor interferes with results. People die as they get older. Therefore, you test survivors and you get healthier and healthier population because the weaker ones have died off.

Despite the problems with testing, there is enough evidence from Dr. Schaie's and many other studies to draw general conclusions about the effects of age on intelligence.

First of all, Raymond B. Cattell and John Horn developed a theory in the 1960s that there are two basic types of intelligence, fluid and crystallized.[5]

Fluid intelligence, also called *performance intelligence,* involves skills, including the coordination of your hands and reacting to a situation where speed is important. It requires quick judgment. It is essentially nonverbal. Although this type of intelligence depends partly on education and experience, it is relatively independent of them and is thought to be most directly related to the functioning of the nervous system.

Crystallized intelligence, also called *verbal intelligence,* involves the ability to use habits of judgment based on experience in order to solve problems. These habits have been "crystallized"—that is, they have taken a definite form—as a result of earlier learning. Crystallized intelligence includes an awareness of terms and concepts reflected in tests of general information and a knowledge of specific fields such as science and mathematics. Although strongly related to educational level and environment, this type of intelligence is, in part, dependent on fluid intelligence. It doesn't involve speed and tends to hold up very well.

It is with fluid or performance intelligence that problems may arise as one gets older since there is a slowing of messages between nerve cells as we age, and this results in slower reaction time. How much of a deficit occurs varies greatly. While a decline in intelligence may include more and more people as time goes by, it does not include everyone! For example, out of one hundred people in their forties, twenty may show an intellectual decline. In their fifties, an additional thirty persons may show a decline, and so on. But there are some who never do manifest a lessening of intellect.[6]

Why? There is no doubt that heredity and health have a lot to do with it, but so does continued intellectual exercise. Learning has been shown recently by a number of researchers working with animals to actually increase the strength of nerve transmission and change the physical properties of nerve endings.[7] They are quite certain that the same holds true for humans and that much of the deficit attributed to aging is actually due to the lack of stimulation of those nerves involved in learning. It is known, from studies conducted at the National Institute of Aging's Baltimore Gerontology Center, that continued intellectual pursuits preserve and even enhance functions in the elderly.

Teaching an old dog new tricks, therefore, aids mental functioning. It also prolongs life. A study of subjects over a twelve-year period

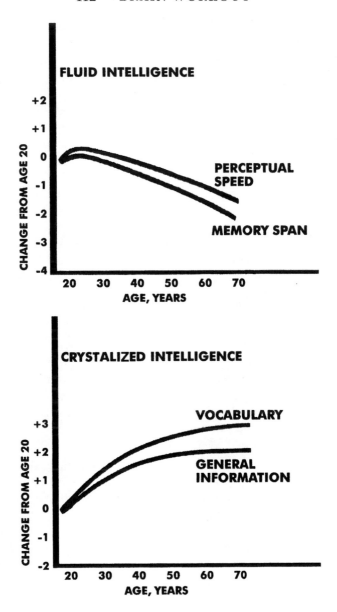

correlated maintenance of intellectual vigor with capacity to survive. Furthermore, aging business executives whose work required sharp intellect show little or no weakening of their nervous systems compared with aging production workers.[8] The inverse is true. Remove stimulation and motivation and you dull cognition and may actually shorten your life.

What can you do to improve your learning, memory and, cognition? First of all, you have to determine what kind of learner you are.

You Are Probably a Sight-Oriented Learner If You:

- are a good speller and can see the words in your mind
- are a strong, fast reader
- would rather read a book than listen to a tape
- doodle while listening to other people lecture
- would rather give a demonstration than a speech
- like art more than music

If this describes you, then when you want to learn something, write it down. Underline or use diagrams and sketching to consolidate information.

Exercise your brain by going to an art museum. Studies have shown that studying paintings aids critical thinking skills.[9] Linda Duke, director of education at the University of Illinois Krannert Art Museum, notes that "intelligent use of visual information, whether derived from art objects, laboratory phenomena, maps, performances, computer screens, or television, is imperative in modern life." Indeed, visual literacy is more relevant than ever before, added Philip Yenawine, a University of Illinois scholar, because "the technology and ability to produce images in large numbers is moving faster than our interest in and ability to study its effects."

You Are Probably a Hearing-Oriented Learner If You:

- often talk to yourself while reading or trying to learn something
- are easily distracted by noise
- find writing difficult and are better at telling what you have to express
- can spell better out loud than in writing
- remember and like to tell jokes
- like music more than art

If you find you are better at processing information by listening to it, use a tape recorder and read what you want to remember or do into the tape. Then play it back.

You Are Probably a Movement-and-Touch-Oriented Learner If You:

- speak slowly
- touch people to get their attention
- stand close to someone when talking or put a hand on the other person
- use a finger when reading
- gesture a lot
- have trouble remembering geography unless you have actually been there
- like to act things out
- learn by manipulating and doing

If you are this type of learner, you will do best by actually acting out or doing whatever you are trying to learn.

After you have determined the easiest way for you to learn, you can consider the relationship between concentration, attention, alertness, memory, and organization.

Concentration, by definition, means to bring one's efforts and faculties to bear on one thing. When you pay *attention,* you are observant or watchful. When you are *alert,* you are vigilant and ready for action, and when you *organize,* you arrange things in a systematic manner. You use all of the above to record and recall memories.

The following exercises will help you exercise these wonderful capabilities of your brain.

Practice Your Powers of Observation

How much do you see without perceiving? There are many things common to our daily life that we do not really register in our minds, or if we do, we cannot recall. Just think of the varied stories eye-witnesses give when asked to describe the scene of an accident. The following test exercises your powers of observation:

1. On a caduceus, the staff carried by the god Hermes and used as an emblem of the medical profession, how many snakes are there below the wings?
2. On a flat map of the world, which continent is to the left of South America and which is to the right?

3. Whose picture is on a ten-dollar bill and what building is on the back?
4. Is the green light on top or bottom on the traffic light?
5. Which stripe is on top of the American flag, the red or white?
6. The Italian flag's colors are green, red, and white. In which order are they, from left to right?
7. On which side does a bride stand at the altar?
8. What are the top and bottom numbers on a fever thermometer?
9. How many nails on a dog's paw?
10. How many points are there on the maple leaf Canada uses on its flag?

Now, to continue to exercise your powers of observation, observe common things in your environment and make up your own quizzes for your family, friends, and/or co-workers. It's fun and will increase your ability to gather information from the world around you.

- How many keys are there on your key ring?
- What color is your postman's hair?
- How many steps are there between two floors in your home.

Speed Up Your Observation Powers

Take a timer and test how long it takes you to circle each arrow that points straight up in the air.

←→↑↓↖↗↑↙↘←→↑↓↖↗↙↘←→↑↓↖↗↙↘↑↑

↑↓↖↗↙↘↑→←↓↑↖↗↙↘→↑↓↖↗↙↘←↑↓↖↑↖

←→↑↖↓↗↙↘←↑↑↓↖↗↙↘←↑↓↖↗↙←←↑↓↓↖↑

↑↓↖↓↑↙↘←→↑↓→↘↑←→↗↙↘↓←→↘↖↑↑↓

Answers: 1. Two snakes are wound around the staff. 2. Australia is on the left and Africa is on the right. 3. Alexander Hamilton and the Treasury building. 4. Bottom. 5. Red. 6. Green, white, and red. 7. The right. 8. 92 and 6. 9. Five. 10. Eleven.

There are seventeen up arrows and you should be able to circle them in twenty seconds. Now, try to find all the arrows that are left-angled. (Hint: There are nine.) Do it within fifteen seconds.

How many left-angled arrows are there really? You've learned another lesson: Trust your own observations!

Attention Getter

There can be no learning without attention. Those who work in cognitive rehabilitation have found that it is not just memory that is a problem, but getting patients to pay attention. The centers are using computers with dots that flash on the screen as an exercise. You can use the traditional child's game of slap-the-hand. Place your hand on a table and have your partner randomly try to tap it before you withdraw it. Your partner should make the attempts irregularly so that you will not know when the tap is coming. This will help not only your attention but your reflexes.

Picking Out Priorities

Take a newspaper or magazine article, cover the headline, and read the article. Write your own headline and then summarize in one paragraph the most important material in that article. You should do this for at least one article every time you read a magazine or newspaper. It is really one of the best cognition exercises available because it helps you identify and organize important material.

Increase Your Arousal Level

Ask yourself how important is it? Lee Iococca, the man who saved the Chrysler car company, says that if it is important, you will remember it. If you are trying to learn something or trying to remember to do something, you first have to convince yourself of its importance. Why do you really want to remember or learn? It is like driving in a car and trying to remember your directions to a certain point. You'll find that the driver who must concentrate on the car and road will remember better than the passenger in the front seat.

You can also increase your mental awareness by proper breathing and exercise (see chapter 4).

Employ Your Sense of Smell for Alertness

Use your sense of smell to increase vigilance. In order to learn, you have to be alert. Recent experiments showed that certain fragrances, such as peppermint and lily of the valley, can have a stimulating effect. University of Cincinnati researchers tested subjects with tasks related to computer monitors. These activities are similar to those of air traffic controllers or long-distance drivers. These jobs require that a high level of vigilance be maintained. At first the subjects accomplished a high level of accuracy but as time went on, their performance deteriorated, as normally happens.[10]

In the experiment, professors William Dember and Joel Warm of the Department of Psychology isolated subjects in a booth where puffs of either peppermint, pure air, or flowery lily of the valley fragrance were administered through a mask every five minutes while the subjects tackled a forty-minute computerized vigilance test. The test required the subjects to hit a button on the computer keyboard whenever a particular pattern of lines appeared.

During the first study, subjects receiving whiffs of fragrance detected the test signals 85 percent of the time during the first ten minutes of testing. Those receiving puffs of plain air detected less than 65 percent. Performance dropped for all groups over the course of the testing, but the fragrance groups significantly out-performed the pure-air group throughout the forty-minute vigil.

Another psychology professor at the University of Cincinnati, Raja Parasuraman, conducted a parallel study with peppermint that provided some clues as to how the fragrances produce their effect. That study not only confirmed that peppermint improved performance on vigilance tests, but Parasuraman also detected unique brain-wave patterns in the fragrance group associated with increased alertness.

Don't Let Emotions Interfere

If something is on your mind, write down what is bothering you. This almost magically helps you to concentrate. Also see the relaxation exercises in chapter 12.

Take Notes from Print or from Discussion

You can practice this by taking down the salient points made by a TV talk show guest as an excellent exercise. This encourages you to pay attention to what is important, and writing down the information reinforces it in your memory and exercises your concentration and prioritizing skills.

Organize Your Information

Underline important pieces of information. Make lists. Take notes. Outline. Make up questions about what you are trying to learn. Identify supportive details. Circle the most important words that signal what you wish to learn or remember.

Set a List of Weekly and Daily Goals

Give the time and date by which you wish the goals to be attained.

Rehearse, Rehearse, Rehearse

As was pointed out in other chapters, repetition creates changes in the cells, and if you want to learn something or perform better, keep rehearsing.

Keep a Diary

By recording what has happened during the day, you are evaluating what occurred. Reminiscing on paper has been found to be an excellent way of exercising mental functions. It is also a good emotional outlet.

Learn a New Language

There are many opportunities to learn a foreign language today, no matter what your age or where you live. There are adult schools, colleges, cassettes, computer programs, and cable TV courses.

Why should you make the effort?

Learning a new language is one of the best brain builders available. Researchers at Montreal Neurological Institute used the PET scan to investigate whether a second language "lights up" the same area of the brain as a first language does. The subjects were normal bilingual people who had learned a second language after the age of five years. Comparison of the blood flow in the brain when repeating words in their second language and repeating words in their native language yielded only a single significant blood flow change—in the putamen, a group of cells in the center of the brain. This means there are increased demands imposed on the brain by speaking a second language.[11]

Although just how language processing is done by your brain is still being debated among neurolinguists, neurologists, psycholinguists, and a host of other specialists, all agree that it is a marvelous and complicated phenomenon. For more than one hundred years, it was believed that language function was located in the left hemisphere, particularly in two key sections of the left-front part of the cortex known as Broca's and Wernicke's areas, named respectively after two nineteenth-century neurologists. They discovered that lesions to these areas caused distinct types of inability to communicate. In Broca's aphasia, associated with lesions in the back of the frontal lobe of the left hemisphere near the area that controls speech, both speech and writing are usually severely affected. The difficulty in speaking is demonstrated in trouble finding a word or certain sounds. Nevertheless, the words are usually employed correctly and what is said often makes sense. In Wernicke's aphasia, associated with lesions farther back in the brain, near the primary sound-receiving area in the left hemisphere, speech frequently is very fluent but meaningless.

Since the observations of Broca and Wernicke, others have found that producing good communication involves many parts of the brain. It is now believed that while various areas may specialize in certain aspects of language, there is a complicated, widespread interchange that occurs among the left and right hemispheres, the motor cortex, and even the deeper structures, including those involved with emotions.[12]

Therefore, by learning a new language, you will be greatly stimulating wide areas of your brain and exercising your memory, speech, and writing centers and generally benefiting your cognitive abilities.

Turn Off the TV and Read, Read

It is very easy to come home after a tiring day and turn on the TV, but greater benefits to your brain will accrue from reading newspapers, magazines, or books. Reading requires more concentration, and what you are concentrating upon will usually be more nourishing to your brain. Youngsters often try to concentrate on their homework while watching TV. As they soon learn when they see their marks, concentration means focusing on one thing at a time.

Get Enough Sleep

You cannot learn well if you are too tired. If you consider how much our ancestors without electricity slept—nine to seven hours—it may be that we are shortening the time our natural circadian rhythm mandates we should sleep. Overloaded personal schedules and a twenty-four-hour-a-day economy are causing chronic sleep deprivation for millions of Americans, according to leading sleep experts.[13] Sleep is defined as the biological and behavioral state in which humans are normally quiet and relatively unresponsive to external stimuli, traditionally thought of as the time when we end our day of work and activity. What happens when we don't get enough sleep? Disrupted or diminished sleep can impair concentration, judgment, and reaction time, making our ability to perform even simple tasks more difficult and increasing the chance of being in an accident at home, at work, or while driving.[14] Therefore, before a big test or presentation, you are better off with sufficient sleep so you will be alert for the challenge. And new scientific research builds the evidence that you can "learn" while you sleep. Researchers at the University of Arizona, Israel's Weizmann Institute, and at the U.S. National Institutes of Health report that certain skills practiced during the day can be honed while sleeping.

Avi Karni and Dov Sagi of the Weizmann Institute showed that during sleep human subjects improve at skills learned by repetition and that improvement depends on brain activity of the type that occurs during the REM (rapid eye movement) phase of sleep. Matthew Wilson and Bruce McNaughton of the University of Arizona in Tucson found the nerve activity in the brains of sleeping rats helped to strengthen the animals' spatial memories.[15]

These findings indicate that sleep helps consolidate in your memory those skills you practiced during the day. The Israelis said this includes perceptual learning—the improvement of perceptual skills through practice. This includes acquisition and retention of procedural knowledge such as "habits" or "how to" memories.

Learn to Use a Computer

Learning to use computers is excellent for your brain. You have to coordinate hand and eye, follow directions, and react quickly. Computer games are being used in most cognitive rehabilitation centers for those very reasons. Computers have come down in price and are within the means of most households. By learning to use a computer, you will not only exercise your brain, but you will receive a psychological lift because you have joined the Computer Age. You *can* learn the computer at any age, and, in fact, many hospitals are training their older volunteers to use computers to help with the input and output of information. There are also a lot of other computerized learning programs available at local adult schools and colleges. Unlike human teachers, computers have infinite patience and can be available whenever you need them.

Play Games

The game is a basic phenomena that includes challenge, interest, and fun. As mentioned above, video games are very useful, especially those requiring answers to questions or instant reactions to hit a target. Bridge and chess are excellent games to pursue because they require memory and judgment. Crossword puzzles and jigsaw puzzles are also excellent, the former for word recall and the latter for spatial judgments.

Set New Challenges

• Figure out what you really want and then develop the skills to get it!

• Make a list of your objectives for the next year and the next five years. Study the list and then write down how you believe you can meet those aims. The next chapter will help you with the methods.

Learning new things as an adult not only enhances your skills and keeps your knowledge up to date, it gives you a feeling of mastery and heightened self-esteem. You then have the confidence to continue to build your brain power and to interact with younger, high-powered people.

8

Free Your Creativity

Creativity is good for your brain. It involves the release of tension, provides gratification, and generally aids your ability to cope. Expressing yourself creatively literally changes the chemistry of your brain and body.

Creativity is not limited to painting, writing a novel, or to scientific innovations. It involves your ability to use your brain to change, renew, and recombine aspects of your life. Creativity means sensing the world with vigor and making new use of what you have perceived.

Children are naturally creative because everything is novel to them. Unfortunately, our school systems follow predetermined paths, and those who want to make new trails run into many booby traps.

Creativity is not encouraged in adults, either. True creativity, however, is not constrained by age. Our youth-oriented society rarely considers the possibility that people past sixty-five years of age can produce creative solutions or products. The *New York Times* carried a front-page article about a New York City woman, Bessie Doenges, who obtained her first literary agent at the age of ninety-four. She was writing a column every week for the newspapers and decided it was time to start writing books: "It seems to be a reason for living—to get this down," she was quoted as saying.

Creativity fights what some have termed "psycho-sclerosis"—the hardening of attitudes many identify with old age; it helps revive childlike pleasures, such as wonder, curiosity, playfulness, and imagination; it allows an adult to find new solutions and new enjoyment of their present stage in life.

Creativity does not necessarily require high intelligence and good marks. On the contrary, high IQ may inhibit the inner resources of the individual because of rigid self-criticism or rapid learning of cultural standards. The great ability to deduce according to the laws of logic and mathematics makes for disciplined thinkers, but not necessarily creative ones. Therefore, it is not surprising that most creative people dislike school. As pointed out earlier in this book, Albert Einstein did so poorly in school, for example, that teachers thought he was slow.

In a narrow-minded, unimaginative environment, being creative can be a disadvantage. A question, which has intrigued researchers for centuries, is: Does being a creative individual and "different" from other people cause emotional problems, or do the emotional problems fuel creativity?

Neuroscientists as well as psychotherapists are spending a lot of time trying to find the answer. There is evidence that in most of us, the right hemisphere of our brains is the fount of creativity while the left is more logical. The left side is concerned with the spoken language, right-side body controls, numbers skills, written language, reading and reasoning, and our own sense of who we are. The right side makes sense of experiences, finds patterns in events, and responds emotionally. The right side is involved in left body control, music awareness, three-dimensional forms, and art awareness. Imagination, intuition, and creativity are right there, waiting for you to draw upon them.

Your right and left brain communicate through the corpus callosum, a thick bunch of "telephone" wires—nerve fibers—that join the two halves of your brain.

Before-and-after studies in problem solving show that a good connection between the two brain hemispheres enhances the ability to come up with answers to problems, which often require both intuitive and intellectual faculties.

There are neuroscientists who believe that in Western society we emphasize the left side of the brain, favoring our scientists and engineers. In fact, there are now courses to teach engineers to make greater use of the right side of their brains so they can have more fun and intuition and see "global pictures" instead of just parts.[1]

Blair Justice, Ph.D., a professor of psychology at the University of Texas School of Public Health in Houston, says the creative process naturally involves exploring feelings and learning more about oneself: Soul-searching and self-knowledge are important for mental health.

James Pennebaker, Ph.D., a psychology professor at Southern Methodist University in Dallas and the author of *Who Gets Sick? How*

Beliefs, Moods, and Thoughts Affect Your Health, says that blood samples taken before and after students had written about emotional experiences showed increased activity among immune system components, such as T cells.

Writing about feelings releases stress. Dancing is also beneficial. The rhythm and movement not only provides exercise but also increases production of certain hormones in the brain, including norepinephrine. Low levels of norepinephrine are associated with depression.

Studies have shown that music and beautiful vistas stimulate release of endorphins, the pain-relieving substances in the brain.

You don't have to be crazy to be creative, but the studies have shown a similarity between certain brain chemicals in schizophrenics and in artists and other creative individuals.

Thorton Sargent, a biophysicist at Lawrence Berkeley Laboratory of the University of California, for instance, is tracing the disposition of amphetamine-like molecules closely related to dopamine in the brain.

"The thing that is really intriguing is that there is evidence of hallucinatory activity caused by some of the molecules similar to that experienced by schizophrenics," Sargent says. "We have found that some of these molecules actually concentrate in the retina. This high concentration of trace material found in the retina [imaging-receiving cells at the back of the eye] suggest that visual hallucination may actually originate in the retina."[2]

Dr. Jon Karlsson, an eminent psychiatrist at Napa State Hospital in California, also is investigating whether the same process that produces the creative "high" in an artist can also produce the disrupted perceptions and behavior experienced by the schizophrenic.[3]

Chances are that scientists will ultimately discover that the difference between schizophrenia and creativity may merely be in the levels of the same neurotransmitters in their brains.

Neurotransmitters are known to be a major factor in another mental illness also associated with creativity—depression. Dr. Karlsson and many other researchers have pointed out that some of the world's great modern poets, writers, and artists have taken their own lives in fits of dejection. Charles Darwin, according to the California research, had classic symptoms of manic-depression, in which there are periodic mood swings, from hyperactivity to the depths of despair.

Schizophrenia and depression, of course, have to do with how an individual perceives the world. In the former, the incoming stimuli may be too strong and/or disorganized; in the latter, the input is too weak. In the former, the neurotransmitter dopamine is believed to be involved; in the latter, the neurotransmitter epinephrine is relevant.

Many neuroscientists, particularly neuropsychiatrists, maintain that the famous writers and artists who were mentally ill created despite of the abnormal brain chemistry, not because of it. Frederic F. Flach, M.D., a New York psychiatrist, is one who has made a specialty of studying the creative process. He maintains: "You do have to be free enough of the norms to see something in a fresh way, and you have to be able to ignore the criticism of the establishment, but usually neuroses and psychoses impede rather than help creativity." He adds that creativity does often follow a period of depression. By its very nature, depression is associated with endings, and because each ending involves starting over, depression can lead to a new beginning.[4]

While there is much yet to be learned about the fascinating correlation between the neurochemistry of mental illness and creativity, what we are concerned with in this book is increasing the potential of the "normal" brain. Creativity is one of the most marvelous products of the "fit brain."

How can you increase your creativity?

There are two major concepts about creativity among neuroscientists. Some believe that almost everyone is capable of great creative achievement, but the potential is used by only a few geniuses among us. Others believe that creativity is something with which you are born and cannot be taught nor instilled by training, any more than left-handedness, perfect pitch, or 20/20 vision can. But, while the neurochemical and psychological processes of creativity may be debated, there is no doubt that there are techniques you can master to develop your own novel ways of using your brain, no matter what your age.[5]

The following are exercises to determine which side of your brain you use most.

Left and Right Brain

Ask a friend or relative a question and observe whether he or she looks to the right or left when answering. If the person looks to the left, he or she is giving you an intuitive or creative answer. If the glance is to the right, that person is giving you a logical or thought-out response.

Throughout art history, the most important work is usually located

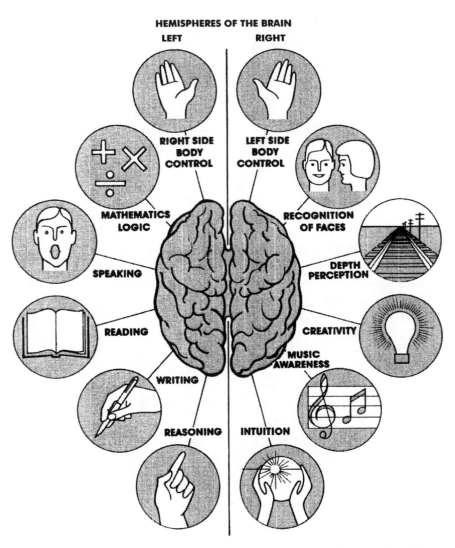

HEMISPHERES OF THE BRAIN
LEFT   RIGHT

RIGHT SIDE   LEFT SIDE
BODY   BODY
CONTROL   CONTROL

MATHEMATICS   RECOGNITION
LOGIC   OF FACES

SPEAKING   DEPTH
                           PERCEPTION

READING   CREATIVITY

                           MUSIC
                           AWARENESS
WRITING

REASONING   INTUITION

in the right half of the picture. Neuroscientists, explaining what the artists have instinctively known, say that when you view a painting, the right hemisphere of your brain is selectively activated and entices your attention toward the left part of the picture. Pictures that correct for this imbalance by having the more important content on the right side are considered the more esthetically pleasing.[6]

There are brain researchers who maintain that geniuses in our society subordinate the normally dominant left hemisphere, the seat of logic and linear thinking, to the right hemisphere, the site of intuition and dreaming. Great art, it is now conjectured, may be the product of the artist's right brain–left brain interplay.

A Simple Test of Your Dominant Brain Hemisphere

Clap your hands once and hold the position.

Which hand is on top? A right-handed person will normally have his or her right hand on top as the hand that took the initiative. The left hand will be the passive one. Neurologists say that occasionally people who are right-handed will use their left hand as the dominant one, but it is rare.

If you are right-handed, it is the left side of your brain that is dominant. If you are left-handed, it is your right side that is dominant. If you use your right hand all the time but when you applaud—that is, your left hand is on top—you may be naturally left-handed but your use of your right hand was encouraged by your parents. And some people can use both hands almost equally well.

Another Test of Your Handedness

Write the following:

> I am looking at my hand as it is writing. Am I left-handed or right-handed? If I am right-handed, is my wrist straight as I am writing? If I am left-handed, is my wrist curled or straight as I am writing?

Dr. Jerre Levy of the Department of Psychology at the University of Chicago found that almost all right-handers keep their wrists straight because their language processing emanates from the opposite (left) side of their brains.[7] When a lefty curls his wrist to write in almost an upside-down hand position, it indicates that he is using the left side of his brain for language processing, just as the straight-wristed right-hander is doing. However, the lefty who keeps his wrist straight while writing is using the opposite side of his brain, the right, for language processing. The curled wrist position, therefore, is a biological marker that indicates that the side of the brain being used for language processing is on the same side as the writing hand.

In any case, using your nondominant hand frequently is exercise for your brain. Proof is that when people's dominant side of their brains are injured by trauma or a stroke, they often can train themselves to let the opposite side of their brains take over and learn to use their non-dominant hand very well.

Dr. Levy and her colleagues have reported that those who use the same side of their brain to write and to process language have a slower reaction time when tested, although there has been some controversy about this observation. Current theory is, nevertheless, that in most people, the right side of the brain is the reservoir of creativity. (Exercises to stimulate the right side of the brain are given later in the chapter.)

Since, as we mentioned earlier, our society in general and our schools in particular subvert creativity, how can we release our natural ability to innovate?

Mining our own preconscious may be one answer.

Dr. Flach points out that psychotherapy can be a creative act because it uncovers new relationships among new and old data in an individual: "The person who is creative has the ability to envision things in different ways; to have a fresh outlook. But the source of a creative idea is not the conscious or the subconscious but the preconscious."[8]

According to Dr. Flach and other psychoanalysts:

To be conscious means to be aware and to have a perception of oneself, one's acts, and one's surroundings.

The preconscious includes all ideas, thoughts, past experiences, and other memory impressions that with effort can be consciously recalled.

The subconscious is a state in which mental processes take place without conscious perception.

Dr. Flach explains that when we are conscious, we are aware of our surroundings but we are limited by the pedestrian restrictions of conscious language. In our subconscious, our feelings are buried so deeply that they are inaccessible. Our painful past experiences and emotions are locked up. In our preconscious we have things close to the surface. It's our computer data center where we put things together—memories, fantasies, and the vibrations we pick up from other people. We are in touch with ourselves.

The preconscious can be tapped under hypnosis. Individuals are asked to observe various objects in a room and then recall them. Then, when under hypnosis, which opens up the preconscious, they are able to recall nearly ten times the number of details as they did at the conscious level.

The creative process itself is said to be a way for the artist to master the internal conflicts—disturbing images that are in the subconscious and preconscious as well as the conscious. Dr. Flach maintains the major need to create, however, is the drive toward finding oneself: "Creativity is not just a product or an act but a way of viewing and reacting in new and constructive ways. You have to adapt and readapt to your environment at home, at work, and in your relationships. You also have to trust your intuition. Intuition is quite different from impulsiveness. It involves perceiving something along preconscious routes frequently by passing ordinary logic. It is often an artist's or writer's intuition that makes masterpieces."

While the psychotherapists, neuroanatomists, and neurochemists are trying to understand the physiologic factors underlying the cognition that produces creativity, they agree that there is little doubt that most of us have a potential for creativity that we do not fully develop.

How You Can Increase Your Creativity

The following are basic exercises that have been shown to stimulate areas of your brain that are known to be involved in creativity.
- Name as many different breeds of dogs you can.
- Fill in: Her eyes were as green as   ,
- Within three minutes, write every word you can think of that begins with Y. If you can compete against someone, so much the better. Thinking while competing is a good exercise for the real world.
- Make as many different things from the circles and squares below as possible.

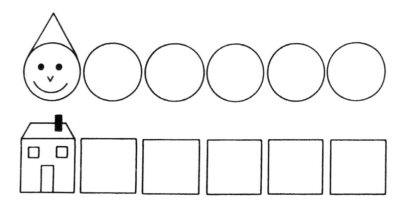

"Punnies"—Creative Humor

Humor has been shown to be one of the best medicines for mind and body. Here's an exercise to help you stir up your creativity. A pun is the humorous use of a word where it can have different meanings. The following is a list of words. Make up your own funny definition. For example:

Good-Bye   A bargain

There is no right or wrong answer. Some other people's definitions are given for your amusement:

Bartender	Soft pole
Kidnap	Sleeping goat
Youthful	Youngster who ate too much
Neighborhood	Local thug
Friendship	Pal's boat
Despair	Set of twins
Makeshift	Change directions

You can make up a list on your own or with friends. It is not only fun, it is a good workout for your brain.

Write a One-Page Letter to Yourself from Someone Else

Let the words flow. You don't have to show it to anyone so have fun with it. It will stir up your creativity and at the same time give you some insight into what you really think of yourself. Some suggestions for the author of your letter:
- a famous person in history, such as Winston Churchill or Samson
- your favorite movie or TV star
- a character from a favorite novel or nonfiction book
- the president of the United States

Uncover and Rid Yourself of Creativity Inhibitors

The process where you talk about yourself and delve back into your experiences with a friend or a therapist may unleash your creativity. Psychotherapy can uncover new facts or new relationships among new and old data and rid you of inhibitions caused by people and circumstances you faced in the past—that teacher who told you that you were inadequate or the need to earn money for necessities. Reminiscing can give you a fresh outlook.

Play with Blocks

When trying to solve a problem, imagine you are a child again, playing with blocks. You experiment, trying to construct something. Piling some blocks here and some there. You will not be upset if the pile falls over. You try another method of building. You learn by experience. Pretend the elements that make up your problem are blocks. Try to rearrange them until you have a structure that pleases you.

The following are techniques developed by New York's Dr. Flach, Dr. Morris Stein, and many psychologists and psychiatrists to help people free themselves from the restrictions of routine and to use their innate creativity to develop new projects, find solutions to problems, and to adapt to change.[9] You can use the following steps in your own life for whatever it is you wish to create.

Prepare Yourself. Do as much reading and talking about whatever it is you wish to create—a solution, a picture, a new approach to a business. Do your homework.

Incubate. We all want quick solutions, but when the answers don't come right away, put the thought aside. Let it simmer in your subconscious. At a later point, perhaps a week or month later, there will be a breakthrough.

Illuminate. In cartoons, this is depicted by a light bulb over the head. It is the point when the breakthrough occurs; something pops into your head and you say, "Ah, that's a good idea."

Test. Now that you've come up with the creative solution, you have to apply it. If there is a new way to handle your marriage, for example, put it into practice. If you have a new way of creating a sculpture, do it. Dr. Flach says that nobody gets the Nobel Prize for a new idea. They get it for testing the idea and showing it works.

Distance Yourself. You can do this merely by changing the room in which you are working or your clothes. Take a "mental excursion": think about a pleasant trip you took or a place you'd like to go. Look at pictures far removed from your ordinary interests or work.

Have a Variety of Leisure Pursuits. Don't spend your leisure time at one avocation, such as tennis or watching TV. Get a variety of experiences. Meet new people. Read new books. First of all, leisure should relax you. It is hard to be creative when you are tense. And by avoiding routine—tennis only or TV only—you gain the stimuli of various people and environments and you use a variety of your muscles and talents. Variety is fertilizer for creativity.

Find Security. It is very difficult to be creative if you are worried about survival. You need to find someone on whom you can depend. Anxiety blocks the free flow of creativity.

Don't Play a Role. If you select a role, such as the Man in the Gray Flannel Suit or the Superwoman, you get locked in and can't do things another way.

Choose Your Associates Carefully. If you associate with people who are constantly tearing you down, criticizing you, you won't be able to create.

Don't Be Afraid to Be Alone. If you are to be creative, you need time to listen to your inner self instead of someone or something else. Then you have to decide what it is you want to do. Is it to paint, write, or solve a problem in your life? See the exercise below to help you decide. Start with your goal in the oval. Then make "spokes" of the ways you think you might achieve that goal.

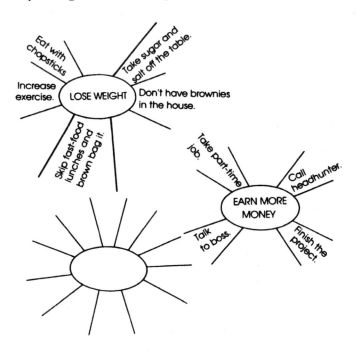

Try to Turn Down Your Motor. You need some inactive and quiet time to let your thought processes work. That means daydreaming. A form of mental activity frowned upon by parents and teachers, it is useful and may open up new channels. You can also reminisce and allow past successes and failures to flow through your mind for reevaluation.

Be Disciplined. It may seem paradoxical, but unstructured environments are not conducive to creativity. You have to have a certain degree of structure in order to be able to create.

Keep a Pencil and Notebook Handy. You can capture fleeting ideas that may later prove to be valuable. You never know what connections may be made between what is novel to you and what you ordinarily have to do.

Find Your Best Time. You are influenced by your biological rhythm. There is a time of day or night when you are at your best. You probably know it, but if you want to make sure, it is probably the time when your body temperature is highest.

Find Your Best Place. Try to remember where you got your best ideas. Some people like to think in a warm bathtub and others while walking or working with their hands.

Write or Tape Your Frustrations. When you are feeling frustrated or tied up in knots and the ideas won't come, write or record what is bothering you. It will help "clear the decks" for action.

Farm Your Brain. Verbalize or write down as many ideas as you can dig out of your brain. Let your mind wander and consider all sorts of solutions. You can help yourself till the fertile soil by making analogies. For example, "I want to paint a better picture but it is like squeezing the last bit of toothpaste from the tube."

Start at the End. Sometimes it is more fruitful to start at the end with the goal you have in mind. The first step is to determine the result you want and then go back to the beginning. Review your present situation, list your options, and think about the best ways you can reach that goal.

Don't Keep Going over the Same Track. If you have a problem you can't solve or a goal you can't meet, stop thinking about it. Let it rest instead of going over it and over it again. Let it "incubate." It's just as if you can't remember a name and it suddenly pops into your mind. The solution, if you let it simmer, may suddenly come.

Defer Judgment. Really listen to your own thoughts, but don't judge your ideas right away. Don't say, "That's foolish" or "That won't work." By offering negative adjectives, you block the flow of ideas.

Keep coming up with solutions no matter how crazy they may sound. Quantity will eventually produce quality.

Don't Be Afraid to Make Mistakes. If you fail, learn what doesn't work. Try a new approach. If you are not failing, you are not being very creative because new trails are unmarked and full of pitfalls. Do not be afraid of failure. We often put off doing something creative— with writers it is called "writer's block"—because we are overwhelmed by the idea of the endeavor or we are afraid of failure. You can help yourself to get started by beginning with just one small part of what you want to do—a paragraph, a phone call, a note. Once you have done the first, you can link it to a second and you are on your way.

Don't Make Excuses. Age, infirmity, and lack of time are frequent reasons given for not being able to create. They are rarely valid. Picasso at age ninety-one, kept art supplies by his bed in case he awoke during the night and had a good idea. He could then capture it on paper. George Bernard Shaw wrote *The Millionairess* in his eighties, and Gabriel Faure's output increased in quantity and quality during his eighth decade of life, even in the face of severe sensory impairment.

Bernice Neugarten, Ph.D., one of the first social scientists to devote her career to the study of aging, observed before a Congressional hearing in the late 1970s: "People fifty or sixty or seventy are doing things today which they would not and could not have done fifty years ago with social or family approval.

"Today, persons of these ages return to school for additional education, begin new careers, marry or remarry, reenter the labor market, retire and travel widely, or devote themselves entirely to leisure pursuit."[10]

9

Food and Supplements to Fuel Your Brain

Did you ever wonder why you were sleepy after a big lunch, or jittery after too many cups of coffee? In such instances, you were aware of what caused the changes in your mental function and mood, but did you know that whatever you eat or drink affects your brain to some degree?

Food fuels your brain and powers its control over your body. Neurotransmitters—those electrochemical messengers sent between nerve cells—are made directly and indirectly from the nutrients you ingest.

What you eat influences production of the hormones needed by your brain to oversee your body functions, and food provides the vitamins vital to its vitality. Your meals provide substances that your brain requires but cannot make, such as glucose and choline.

Your brain's major fuel is glucose—blood sugar—which is derived from foods, primarily starches and simple sugars. It is present at all times in the blood, usually in an amount maintained within quite a narrow range. Studies using the PET scanner trace the mind's workings through chemical "footprints." These studies have shown that the brain's capacity to use glucose remains pretty stable well into old age if we remain healthy.[1]

In contrast, those with Alzheimer's disease, which causes deterioration of the brain and severe memory deficits, show significant impairment in the use of glucose, particularly in the inner areas of their brains.

Although there is a great deal of controversy among scientists about the effects of ingested foods on the brain, no one denies that you can change your ability to think and your mood by what you eat.

Sugar's Effect on the Brain

Let's consider sugar first, since it is the major fuel. Directly after you eat a meal, your glucose level rises. Then, your pancreas secretes insulin to help move sugar into the cells, and your glucose level drops. However, if your blood sugar falls to lower than normal levels following a meal your brain doesn't get enough and sends out distress signals.

There are two basic types of low blood sugar:

Reactive Hypoglycemia, which occurs about two to four hours after eating, especially if the meal was high in carbohydrates. As the blood sugar drops, the person suddenly experiences dizziness, fatigue, weakness, nervousness, and heart palpitations. These symptoms are not unlike those of an acute anxiety attack. They are the result not of the low blood sugar, however, but of too much of the hormone epinephrine (adrenalin), which is sent to signal the liver to make more glucose.

Fasting Hypoglycemia, which occurs more slowly and is more rare and serious. It occurs during the night or before breakfast and can be associated with conditions such as alcoholic intake, misuse of diabetic drugs, or a serious underlying disorder, such as an insulin-secreting tumor or liver disease.

We all can suffer from hypoglycemia if we suddenly binge on high-calorie carbohydrate meals after eating little throughout the day.

If you do not have a medical condition that causes hypoglycemia but you do have minor problems with maintaining your blood sugar levels (evidenced by waking with headaches) and wish to avoid distressing your brain with too little fuel, try the following sensible eating pattern:

• Avoid sweets, pastries, and sugar-laden drinks such as colas and cocoa.

• Forgo alcoholic beverages that can cause the blood sugar to drop.

• Instead of two or three meals a day, eat six small high-protein meals. By eating frequently, you eat less each time so that rather than have three wide swings upward and downward in your blood sugar, you can maintain it on a more even keel.

• A protein snack at bedtime may avoid your waking up with a headache caused by low blood sugar.

Another problem due to sugar is *diabetes,* a condition in which blood sugar levels are too high, resulting in damage to the brain and body. Type II diabetes, which occurs in adulthood, can often be prevented and/or combated merely by diet, weight loss, and exercise. Type I diabetes, which is more serious, requires medication to control blood sugar.

Researchers have found that when there are high levels of sugar in the blood—whether or not the patient suffers from diabetes—the severity of brain damage is increased when the supply of blood to the brain is insufficient. In studies of stroke patients, it was found that those with higher blood-sugar levels had more permanent nerve and brain damage than those with lower levels.[2]

Sugar levels in your blood affect not only your brain cells and blood vessels but your ability to think.

Studies done with adults show meals with high sugar levels not only make them sluggish but interfere with their concentration. Dr. Bonnie Spring of Harvard University found that adults had difficulty performing a simple speech test after eating a sherbetlike high-carbohydrate snack. The decline was especially marked for those over forty. Her tests also showed differences in the way men and women felt after eating the snack; women had a more pronounced reaction and reported feeling lethargic and sleepy, while men simply reported feeling calmer.[3]

So, overloading the blood with sugar can cause a paradoxical drop in blood-sugar levels. Skipping meals can also cause blood-sugar levels to be too low for the brain. Dr. Ernesto Pollitt of the University of Texas worked with a group of children and had half of them skip breakfast while the other half ate a meal of waffles and syrup, milk, and orange juice. By late morning, those who ate breakfast made fewer errors solving problems than the children who skipped breakfast.[4]

Choline—The Memory Food Substance

There is a tremendous concentration of research concerning another element in the diet, choline. This is a substance that is found either alone or as part of lecithin and the B-vitamin complex. Choline is in fish, meats, egg yolks, soy products, oatmeal, rice, peanuts, and pecans. It is taken from the digestive tract by the blood and carried to the brain, where it becomes acetylcholine, a neurotransmitter (a messenger between nerves). The nerves that produce acetylcholine are believed to undergo degeneration and to be a cause of the brain dysfunction in Alzheimer's. Acetylcholine is also believed to be involved in other memory problems commonly associated with aging.

Researchers are pursuing the idea that the impairment of the brain's system for using choline in certain diseases and in old age may be prevented or minimized with choline-based materials added to the diet. There has been an effort to increase the building blocks of acetylcholine by increasing lecithin, the normal source of choline, in our diet. Lecithin, from the Greek meaning "egg yolk," is found in large amounts in egg yolks and is commercially isolated from eggs, soybeans, and corn. It is a widely used antioxidant in food. It is known that purified lecithin, which is more concentrated than that sold in health food stores, raises blood levels of choline, but as yet, there are not definitive studies on the benefits of lecithin.

Scientists know that as we age, the capability of transferring information from one cell to another or to a large target organ is markedly reduced. In part, this is due to the amount of acetylcholine and in part to the ability to use what is there.

An enzyme, N-acetyltransferase, helps produce acetylcholine. One of the most consistent neurochemical findings is the reduced activity of this enzyme in the normal-aged human, and its very marked weakness in the brains of Alzheimer's victims. This causes reduced production of acetylcholine.[5] Pharmaceutical researchers are trying to find a way to either increase acetylcholine production by:

• increasing the building blocks of acetylcholine—lecithin and choline;

• inhibiting acetylcholine destruction; or

• directly stimulating the receptors in the brain for choline by sending in a compound that imitates it.

When mice were fed choline-enriched diets over a period of several months, the type of memory deficits typically seen in old mice did not occur. It appeared that prolonged dietary choline treatment somehow enabled the mice to form new long-term memories more efficiently than old mice not on the diet.[6]

In humans, thus far, a choline-enriched diet—meat, fish, dairy products, and grains—has not seemed to help those suffering from moderate to severe memory problems. But researchers are studying the long-term effects of supplements of choline and lecithin, and trying to find pharmaceuticals that may enhance their benefits for brain function.

The Meaning of Aminos

Amino acids derived from the proteins we eat are the starting materials for our brain's chemical messengers, the neurotransmitters. Diets deficient in protein have been reported to cause permanent damage to the intelligence of the young and to affect the memory and cognition of the elderly.[7] Of the twenty amino acids that go into building the millions of proteins in your body, nine cannot be manufactured by your body in sufficient quantities to sustain growth and health and must be obtained from your diet. These are called *essential amino acids* because they are *essential* for maintaining good health.

Your brain is almost completely regulated by amino acids, and their journey from your plate to your head depends on the content of your meals, your physical condition, your activity, and your environment. When you eat a meal of meat, beans, or any other protein-containing food, digestive enzymes in your stomach and small intestines break apart the protein molecule into "free" amino acids and into small bunches of amino acids, called *peptides,* strung together head to tail. Your liver then controls the distribution of amino acids in your blood. As the amino acids move through your bloodstream, your body selects the particular amino acid building blocks it needs for its organs and its functions. That steak you ate, therefore, may become part of your nails or the muscle of your big toe, or it may go to your brain to help get this information you are reading right now across your brain cells.

Your brain uses amino acids to produce enzymes, the "workers" that convert raw materials into useful products. The enzymes, in turn, use amino acids to manufacture chemical brain messengers—neurotransmitters—such as dopamine to help you move and serotonin to calm you down. Each of your brain's neurotransmitters has its own personal enzyme.

Think of a neurotransmitter in your brain as a sentence. The amino acids are the "words" that are strung together in a certain order to form the "sentence." Each sentence, or neurotransmitter, carries a particular message between nerve cells in your brain.

The neurotransmitter sentences are constructed in two ways:

1. directly from the amino acids in the protein you eat
2. indirectly, by causing insulin to be released from your pancreas, which then draws amino acids from your blood and tissues

There are natural, daily fluctuations in amino acid levels in your blood,[8] but the content of your meals can cause major changes in blood and brain levels of these powerful substances and thus affect your thinking, mood, and behavior.

Amino acids are extremely powerful in small doses and are versatile in changing roles, depending upon where they are used in the body. It is not surprising, therefore, that one of the hottest areas in pharmaceutical research today involves amino acids. The fact that amino acids are derived from foods, however, does not mean they are harmless and should be taken lightly. The amino acid levels in your body are exquisitely balanced. By overloading your system with one you can affect the levels of others, which may produce serious adverse effects on your body and brain.[9]

A tremendous amount of research is now in progress to determine how amino acids affect brain function and behavior. Literally thousands of scientific papers are presented each year on the subject. The following describes some of the findings concerning amino acids and the brain.

Tyrosine

Tyrosine is not considered an essential amino acid because it can be manufactured by the body from another amino acid, phenylalanine.

Tyrosine is a building block for the nerve messengers epinephrine and norepinephrine as well as for the thyroid hormones and melanin, the skin and hair pigment. Norepinephrine and epinephrine are neurotransmitters involved in strong emotions and alertness. Thyroid hormones are necessary for normal metabolism of food and also strongly influence the brain and behavior.

Dr. Alan J. Gelenberg, a psychiatrist at Harvard Medical School, reported that some depressed patients who took tablets of tyrosine, in addition to their regular diet, improved. However, the tyrosine provided solely by a high-protein diet did not have the same benefit.[10]

The Tryptophan Trip

Tryptophan, another amino acid, was first isolated from milk in 1901. It is believed to work in partnership with tyrosine to produce the brain chemicals serotonin, dopamine, and norepinephrine. The theory is that nerve cell communication by these powerful brain chemicals can be affected by the availability of tryptophan and tyrosine. Since these two amino acids are supplied by the diet, the possibility is also considered that diet-induced alterations in blood levels of tryptophan and tyrosine can affect serotonin, dopamine, and norepinephrine, and thus the brain and behavior.

When tryptophan is not available to the body at sufficient levels, there is a worsening of the B-vitamin-deficiency disease pellagra. The condition is manifested by mental and nerve disorders.

Eating carbohydrates raises the level of tryptophan. This is why a warm glass of milk or sugary, starchy foods may work to make you sleepy. Dr. Ernest Hartmann of Tufts University School of Medicine has studied the effects of extra doses of tryptophan on groups of normal people and mild insomniacs. Those who took tryptophan tablets fell asleep sooner. This suggests that eating carbohydrate-rich foods, which raise tryptophan levels, might offer similar relief for those troubled by insomnia.

Dr. Michael Yogman of Children's Hospital Medical Center in Boston has also shown the sleep-inducing effects of tryptophan. He reported that babies go to sleep faster when a solution of sugar and tryptophan is added to their bottles, but warned against mothers doing their own experimenting with this amino acid.[11]

Tryptophan, as pointed out, is a building block for the important neurotransmitter serotonin, low levels of which are believed to play a part in depression and sensitivity to pain. Pharmaceutical researchers theorize that tryptophan may be combined with other medications and used as a mild analgesic. In a number of studies, tryptophan in doses of 2 to 3 grams daily, raised the pain thresholds in patients suffering from chronic facial pain and dental pain.[12] It has also been used as an aid to smokers who wish to quit the habit since it reportedly prevents nicotine-withdrawal symptoms.

Tryptophan is also a building block for another neurohormone, melatonin. Melatonin is believed to be important in the timing of body clocks. Disorders of melatonin levels and rhythms are suggested to play a part in depression, abnormal sleep, Alzheimer's disease, and some age-related dysfunctions.

Tryptophan is also a precursor of niacin, which is a critical helper in many biochemical processes, notably energy metabolism. Lack of it can cause neurological disorders. There is evidence that stress and/or dietary lack of tryptophan may make deficiencies of serotonin and melatonin common.[13]

Over-the-counter tryptophan has been withdrawn from the market. In 1989 and 1990, more than 1,200 cases of eosinophilia-myalgia syndrome (EMS) were reported to the Centers for Disease Control; three patients died. All patients reported use of L-tryptophan supplements before the onset of illness. The most commonly reported symptoms were muscle and joint pains followed by shortness of breath or cough and rash. Fluid retention occurred in half and fever was common. The cause was found to be a contaminant in the tryptophan, not the amino acid itself.[14]

A high-protein diet that contains a lot of tyrosine and tryptophan has been used to try to increase the level of dopamine and serotonin in patients with neurological and psychiatric disorders thought to involve these brain neurotransmitters. Doctors who are investigating the amino acids for this purpose say that thus far it looks promising.[15]

Healing Arginine

Arginine, a nonessential amino acid, is important to the production of urine and is necessary for healing wounds. It is the main component of some products touted as "overnight" diet pills. Arginine affects the secretion of growth hormone, which, in turn, supposedly affects appetite—the rationale for its use in appetite-suppressant pills. In large doses it causes nausea, which may be another explanation for its appetite-suppressing quality.

The Methionine Method

Methionine, an essential amino acid, has been found to have antidepressant effects when metabolized with vitamin B-2 into a compound called S-adenosyl-L-methionine (SAM). In several studies this compound was found to be as effective as some antidepressant drugs now widely used, ameliorating symptoms such as guilt, suicidal thoughts, slowness of movement, work problems, and lack of interest. It was also reported to be more rapid in taking effect than conventional antidepressant drugs, with many patients showing improvement after four to seven days as compared to the ten days to two weeks it usually takes with other medications. Methionine also seems to have no apparent side effects. As of this writing it is being clinically tested in the United Kingdom, Italy, and the United States.[16]

Phenylalanine

The essential amino acid phenylalanine is, along with another amino acid, tyrosine, a building block of the brain messenger norepinephrine, which has to do with memory function as well as with sex drive and appetite.

An inborn metabolic defect in which there is an inability to process the phenylalanine in food (phenylketonuria, or PKU) leads to mental deterioration and eventually death if phenylalanine is not restricted in the diet. A deficiency of or an inability to utilize phenylalanine has also been linked to the destruction of nerve coverings, which then interferes with their transmission of messages, producing incoordination and other problems, like those seen in multiple sclerosis. A partner in the destruction of the nerve coverings, according to some theories, is an inability to utilize vitamin B-12. Therefore, phenylalanine and B-12 given together show promise in the treatment of multiple sclerosis and related diseases. In a four-year study of patients with multiple sclerosis, D-phenylalanine was given with B-12. In varying degrees, the patients experienced a reversal in bladder spasms and the return of muscle control.[17]

Phenylalanine has also been used for weight loss, as an antidepressant, and as an antispasmodic. And the food industry is now injecting eight million pounds of phenylalanine into the food supply each year as part of the sweetener aspartame.

Amino Acid Competition

We have a natural defense system called the blood-brain barrier, a collection of brain cells that act like secret service agents to protect a "head of state" against assassins and hecklers. Constantly on guard, the blood-brain barrier allows only a certain amount of particular types of amino acids to pass through at one time. There is competition within each type of amino acid to get past the barrier and into the brain tissue. Once there is "no more room," because its competitors got there first, the blood-brain barrier prevents other amino acids from entering. For example, high-protein meals fail to increase the level of tryptophan in the brain because the other amino acids are much more abundant in dietary proteins. The competition for access to the brain, then, becomes weighted against tryptophan.[18] Thus, whether an amino acid in your diet will get to your brain depends not only on the concentration of the amino acid in your diet and blood but also on the concentrations of its amino acid competitors.

Recognition of this phenomenon has already shown promise in therapy with Parkinson's disease patients. More than one and a half million Americans suffer from this devastating nervous disorder, which is characterized by involuntary trembling of the limbs and facial muscles, extreme slowness of movement, and muscular rigidity that makes even simple activities like walking or picking up a book difficult. Levodopa, a drug that raises the level of dopamine in the brain, is a treatment that has freed many Parkinson's patients from the prison of the disease, but it often produces side effects that are as bad as the disease.

A number of Parkinson's patients have noted that hot, spicy meals result in violent movements, while meat products or other foods rich in protein make them stiffer and slower. These patients determined that a bland or vegetarian diet causes fewer or less severe symptoms. It was discovered that some amino acids may block the absorption of levodopa from the gut or block its entry into the brain.[19]

Yale Medical School physician Jonathan H. Pincus and his associates gave eleven Parkinson's patients a special diet regimen.[20] They were to eat carbohydrates all day and eat proteins only at night. From the time they awoke until 5:00 P.M., the patients ate no meat, poultry, dairy products, legumes, nuts, or baked goods (which contain milk and eggs). After a short time, nine of the patients "experienced a marked relief of parkinsonian symptoms" as well as a lessening of the side effects often brought on by levodopa.[21] Moreover, eight of these patients were able to reduce their dosage of the medication by an average of 41 percent.

Physicians in private practice who read about the results began trying the new therapy on their own patients and are reporting similar successes. But when the high-protein meal is eaten in the evening to make up for the lack of protein all day, "patients experience an exacerbation of parkinsonian symptoms that can last up to three or four hours," Dr. Pincus and his colleagues pointed out. "Nonetheless, the simple measure of avoiding protein during the daytime is allowing patients who suffer from the side effects of levodopa to enjoy hours of near-normal functioning and independence."[22]

Your Diet and Your Amino Acids

So what should you eat to make sure your brain gets the amino acid building blocks it needs to manufacture neurotransmitters in your brain? Your first priority is a diet sufficient in protein. The word *protein* itself means "of first importance." Customary intake by Westerners is 100 grams of dietary protein. You contribute about 70 grams of self-made protein per day and you lose about 10 grams per day by elimination of waste. That means you have to process 160 grams of protein per day.

High-quality proteins contain the essential amino acids in an available form and in near-optimal proportions. Animal proteins—sometimes called "complete proteins"—such as eggs, meat, fish, poultry, and dairy products, are high-quality proteins.

Vegetarian diets tend to lack one or another of the essential amino acids. For example, most rice is low in lysine, while some legumes are low in methionine but high in lysine. So a meal of rice and beans (legumes) provides a combination of food proteins. Nuts or seeds and legumes also provide complementary proteins. (Soy beans are the only beans that contain all the amino acids.)[23]

Many cultures have made use of these dietary combinations for hundred of years without understanding amino acid metabolism—for instance, the Mexican staples of beans and rice or tortillas. Asians have long mixed rice and bean curd; the East Indians mix rice and lentils. In southeastern United States, the combination of rice and black-eyed peas is common. All of these combinations provide a balanced amount of essential amino acids.

Some vegetable proteins can also be supplemented with a small amount of animal protein. The Chinese use small portions of meat or fish in stir-fried vegetables and rice dishes. Americans also use this technique with dishes such as macaroni and cheese, pizza, and even the common sandwich.

Can you manipulate your amino acid intake to affect your brain? You certainly can, but it is best to do it through diet rather than to dose yourself with amino acids without medical supervision. If you want to calm yourself or fall asleep more easily, eat a meal high in carbohydrates and low in protein, which will raise your brain levels of tryptophan and the neurotransmitter serotonin. Choices for a high-carbohydrate breakfast (not a balanced meal, but one weighted toward raising tryptophan) might include any of the following foods:

pears	pancakes with syrup
pineapple juice	bran muffin

oat cereal   decaffeinated coffee or tea
English muffin and jam

Choices for a high-carbohydrate lunch might include any of the following:

spaghetti   cranberry juice
macaroni   apple pie
fresh green beans   lemon meringue pie
rye bread   decaffeinated coffee or tea
potato pancakes   fruit juice
whole-wheat toast and
    tomatoes

Choices for a high-carbohydrate dinner might include:

fettucini   vegetable casserole
baked potato stuffed
    with vegetables   apricots
barley   cherries
eggplant

If you want to be stimulated, be as sharp as possible, and use your memory, or if you are going to participate in an athletic competition, you can stimulate your norepinephrine, dopamine, and acetylcholine levels by eating a diet rich in protein, especially tyrosine and lecithin (to produce acetylcholine). Choices for a high-protein breakfast might include any of the following:

eggs   meat
cottage cheese   milk
yogurt   caffeinated coffee or tea
fish

Choices for a high-protein lunch might include:

egg salad   soybean products, such as tofu
sliced turkey   chili
cheese   tuna
sliced chicken   caffeinated coffee or tea

Choices for a high-protein dinner might include:

steak	chef's salad
lamb chops	salmon steaks
veal chops	cheese soufflé
pork chops	pizza with cheese
halibut	milk
bluefish	caffeinated coffee or tea

Today you can buy foods that contain sufficient proteins so that, ostensibly, you will have an abundance of amino acids from which to build the neurotransmitters in your body. However, the way you cook your food has a significant effect on its amino acid value. For example, Cornell University researchers investigated the amino acid content of potatoes before and after cooking. Fried potatoes are an increasingly popular item in the supermarket. The researchers found that frying the skin decreased its amino acid content by 45 percent. Frying the inside of the potato, as in french frying, increased its amino acid level by 36 percent. By contrast, baking the potato lowered the amino acid content of the skin by only 5 percent, and baking actually raised the amino acid content of the inside of the potato by 13 percent. The skin of the potato has more amino acids than the inside, so you might bake your potatoes and eat the skin as well as the inside.[24]

The interaction in the brain among diet, amino acids, and neurotransmitters is very complicated and depends on many factors. Psychologist Michael Trulson has questioned the immediate cause and effect of ingesting amino acids and changes in behavior.[25]

He suggests that there is no "simple relationship" between diet and brain function, but that perhaps there is a "lag time." He points out that it takes from ten days to two weeks for antidepressant medication to take effect and that perhaps there is also a delay in the effect of a variety of amino acids on brain function.

As scientists continue their studies, more and more information will emerge. Next to water, protein is the most abundant substance in your body. All of your cells contain protein, and you could not think without the protein in your brain. Amino acids are the building blocks of protein and, thus, of your brain, your body, and your life itself. They are extremely powerful in various combinations. If you are smart, your amino acids made you that way. Treat them with respect.

Working together with the amino acids to keep your brain functioning well are the vitamins in your diet.

Vitamins and Brain Function

Vitamins, which were named for the Latin *vita*, meaning "life," are vital to the proper functioning of the brain and act as helpers for the neurotransmitters. It is believed by many gerontologists that one of the problems with cognition in the elderly is that older patients suffer from subclinical malnutrition.

One researcher has dubbed the condition the "tea and white bread syndrome." He explained that because of physical disability or fear of crime, many solitary older people live on tea and white bread, which keeps a long time. They consequently suffer malnutrition.[26]

Memory problems may also cause malnutrition and vitamin deficiency because victims may forget to take prescribed vitamins or may prepare meals inadequately. Researcher James S. Goodwin, M.D., and his colleagues at the University of New Mexico School of Medicine, writing in the *Journal of the American Medical Association,* reported a correlation between low blood levels of vitamins C, B-12, riboflavin, and folic acid and lower scores on standard tests for memory and nonverbal abstract-thinking ability.

Bs Are Brain Vitamins

Vitamin deficiencies—in particular, deficit of the B vitamins (thiamine, niacin, and B-12)—are relatively common among older people, sometimes due to diet inadequacies and sometimes due to malabsorption. When monkeys were deprived of vitamin B (thiamine), they exhibited a pattern of impairment in learning and in recognition of highly familiar items reminiscent of certain memory deficits shown by patients with brain damage and memory deficits due to alcoholism. Postmortem exams in the B-deficient monkeys showed nerve degeneration all over their brains.

The B vitamins are necessary for good nerve function and appetite. But like other vitamins and the amino acids, self-dosing with large amounts is unwise. Cases have been reported of nerve damage due to excessive intake of B vitamins.

Vitamin B-12

According to number of recent studies, vitamin B-12 (cyanocobalamin) may be important in combating Alzheimer's disease as well as depression and panic disorders. Its promise as a nutraceutical for these conditions apparently lies in its ability to inhibit monoamine oxidase (MAO), an enzyme that works with oxygen to break down brain chemicals involved in movement and mood.

Swedish researchers, who found B-12 levels were low and MAO activity high in Alzheimer's patients, gave a group of Alzheimer sufferers B-12 therapy. The Swedes found the MAO activity in the patients' brains was significantly reduced to apparently normal levels. Pharmaceutical monoamine oxidase inhibitors (MAOI), such as phenelzine sulfate and tranylcypromine sulfate, used in treating depression and panic disorders, are more powerful but are used infrequently because of their potentially serious side effects.

This led the Scandinavians to conclude that vitamin B-12 plays a significant part in Alzheimer's.[27] The Japanese added some confirming evidence. Researchers in the department of neuropsychiatry at Yamaguchi University School of Medicine found giving Alzheimer patients B-12 improved intellectual function scores such as memory, emotional, and communication for a prolonged period.[28] Italian studies have also validated B-12's potential usefulness in the treatment of Alzheimer's.[29]

A number of drugs such as antibiotics and those given to treat gout cause malabsorption of vitamin B-12. Such a deficiency may affect the behavior of healthy people of any age, but it is particularly significant for older persons. Over the age of sixty years, a lack of vitamin B-12 may be responsible for developing neurological symptoms, ranging from tingling sensations, inability to coordinate muscular movements, weakened limbs, and lack of balance, to memory loss, mood changes, disorientation, and psychiatric disorders. Senior citizens may be ingesting enough B-12 with their food but more than one in five older Americans may no longer produce enough stomach acid to separate B-12 from the protein-swallowed food. The vitamin, therefore, does not travel from the stomach to the rest of the body.

Unfortunately, while the treatment for B-12 deficiency is simple and inexpensive, the diagnosis is not. One reason is that it is difficult to detect is that it doesn't show up on a routine blood work yet even a mild deficiency, discernible only with the most sophisticated laboratory tests, can result in neurologic abnormalities.[30] About 30 percent of patients with symptoms of vitamin B-12 deficiency may have apparently normal levels on blood tests, according to researchers at the Department of Neurology at the School of Medicine, the State University of New York, Buffalo. They maintain vitamin B-12 replacement should not be withheld from patients with borderline vitamin B-12 levels, since the consequences of allowing muscle, nerve, and brain damage to worsen clearly outweigh any disadvantage of therapy.[31]

In a review article of seventy-nine studies of subtle B-12 deficiency, researchers concluded that a long list of psychiatric illnesses or symptoms—especially some cases of mood disorder, dementia, paranoid psychoses, violent behavior, and fatigue—have been documented to be caused by vitamin B-12 deficiency. The conclusion was that these conditions are possibly more commonly caused by B-12 deficiency than is currently generally accepted, mostly because of a lack of appreciation of how much serum B-12 level is necessary to protect the brain.[32]

Gastroenterologist Robert Russell, M.D., doing research at U.S. Department of Agriculture's Human Nutrition Research Center on Aging at Tufts University, reports the problem is severe enough and widespread enough to say "vitamin B-12 is probably the single most important nutrient affected by aging."[33]

Foods that are high in vitamin B-12 are liver, meat, milk and dairy foods, and eggs.

Vitamin B-6. A Common Partner

Pyridoxine is another B vitamin for the brain. It helps metabolize protein; aids in the production of red blood cells; and maintains proper functioning of nervous system tissue. Vitamin B-6 is believed to act as a partner for more than one hundred different enzymes. A number of the brain chemicals that send messages back and forth between nerves depend upon it for formation. A deficiency in this vitamin is known to cause depression and mental confusion. Seizures have been observed in human infants made vitamin B-6 deficient inadvertently when they were fed a commercial infant formula in which the vitamin had not been properly preserved. Certain substances that deplete B-6 also produce deficiency seizures. Patients are likely to have a deficiency of B-6 if they are alcoholics, or have burns, diarrhea, heart disease, intestinal problems, liver disease, overactive thyroid, or are suffering the stress of long-term illness or serious injury.

Numerous studies have suggested that many pregnant and lactating women may not get enough vitamin B-6 in their diets, which may affect the vitamin B-6 status of their offspring. This nutrient is an essential co-factor in developing the central nervous system and may influence brain growth and cognitive function. Recent work in animals suggest that vitamin B-6 deficiency during gestation and lactation alters the function of the brain for certain neurotransmitters thought to play an important role in learning and memory.[34]

Nerve problems in the arms and legs common in diabetics may also be associated with B-6 deficiency. Diabetics who experienced nerve symptoms and whose urine contained evidence of B-6 deficiency were given 150 milligrams of the vitamin each day for six weeks. The treatment eliminated symptoms of neuropathy in all subjects. A longer study of six months showed similar results.[35]

Vitamin B-6 also reportedly helps rid the body tissues of excess fluid that causes some of the behavioral and physical symptoms of premenstrual tension.

Older people, especially older women, may need more vitamin B-6 than currently recommended by the government. A three-month study of men and women between the ages of sixty-one and seventy-one broadens the age range of data for setting future RDAs for this nutrient.[36] (The current RDAs are based on the needs of younger adults.) The six women in the study required 1.9 milligrams of B-6 compared to the current RDA of 1.6 milligrams. The men needed 1.96 milligrams, which is equal to the current 2-milligram RDA, leaving no safety margin normally built into an RDA. The findings help to explain why older people repeatedly test more deficient in the vitamin than younger ones. Marginal deficiencies don't produce obvious symptoms and can only be detected through biochemical tests. Since B-6 is important for the proper functioning of the nervous system, a persistently low intake could lead to depression, lethargy, confusion, or nervousness. But these symptoms could also result from several other causes.

Overdosing on B-6 is unwise, however. A study reported in the *New England Journal of Medicine* in 1983 described the loss of balance and numbness suffered by seven young adults who took doses of 2 to 6 grams of pyridoxine daily for several months to a year. Other potential adverse reactions include drowsiness and a feeling of pins and needles in limbs.

Vitamin B-1 Helps to Fuel the Brain

The link between vitamin B-1 (thiamine) and the brain is strong: Our bodies cannot manufacture the vitamin, yet B-1 is needed to process the only fuel the brain can use—the blood sugar glucose. Because of this vital need, the nervous system is particularly susceptible to thiamine deficiency. Thiamine treatment as much as 300 milligrams per day, is used in cases of Wernicke's encephalopathy, an acute brain disorder sometimes called cerebral beriberi. In the early stages there is mental confusion, inability to think of a word, and making up of "facts." As it progresses, there are delusions, loss of memory, loss of balance, and eye problems. In industrialized countries, where this syndrome is associated with thiamin deficiency, the patients are usually alcoholics.

Vitamin B-2. The Liver-and-Milk Vitamin

Riboflavin, also called lactoflavin or hepatoflavin (because milk and liver are its main natural sources) has a high affinity for your brain, which helps explain the long-standing observation that even in severe riboflavin deficiency, its concentration in the brain does not decline appreciably. Vitamin B-2 reportedly fights stress, and its chemical structure is similar to chlorpromazine (Thorazine), the powerful tranquilizer.[37]

Folic Acid

This B-compound vitamin has now been proven to be necessary for the prevention of serious birth defects of the brain and spinal cord. Folic acid may also have an effect on brain function in the elderly. One study found that elderly patients with mental disorders, especially dementia, were three times more apt to have low folic acid than others their age.[38]

Even among a group of healthy older people, those with low folic acid intake scored lower on abstract-thinking ability and memory. Further, even borderline deficiencies have been found to be harmful and daily doses of folic acid supplements—200 micrograms (found in a three-quarter cup of cooked spinach)—have lifted mood and relieved depression.

In another study, a group of 38 patients with minor neurological signs but with depression, fatigue, lassitude, and burning feet and restless leg syndrome (see glossary) were given supplementary folic acid. The burning feet and restless legs syndrome improved during the first three weeks.[39] Their fatigue and depression cleared in about two to three months.

Foods high in folic acid include liver, lentils, dry beans, asparagus, green leafy vegetables, fish, meats, wheat products, and broccoli.

The Antioxidant Vitamins and the Brain

Head trauma, stroke, lung ailments, and other conditions that block the flow of oxygen to the brain cause the release of free radicals—those highly reactive molecules that quickly damage sensitive nerve cells. Neuroscientists have been hard at work trying to determine whether vitamins A and E and other antioxidants—which quickly sop up these free radicals—can protect the brain against them. Dr. S. Goldstein of the University of Arkansas for Medical Sciences, pointed out in the medical journal *Geriatrics* that because nerve cells in the adult human do not replicate as colon and bone marrow cells do, nerve cells must be protected against oxygen damage. "Natural antioxidants such as vitamins C and E and beta carotene, as well as an optimal caloric and protein intake, should be cornerstones of treatment and prevention in the aging patient."[40]

Beta Carotene for the Brain

Eating foods rich in beta carotene, another antioxidant, may protect against memory loss and other loss of neurologic function, according to Dutch researchers. In a study of more than 5,100 people age fifty-five to ninety-five, those who consumed less than 0.9 milligrams per day of beta carotene were almost twice as likely to suffer from cognitive impairment and disorientation and to have difficulty solving problems as those who consumed 2.1 milligrams per day.[41]

Vitamin E and Parkinson's Disease

Major medical institutions in the United States and abroad have been investigating whether vitamin E may prove effective in treating such brain conditions as Parkinson's and Alzheimer's diseases.

A multimedical center investigation of vitamin E with and without the medication selegiline—which inhibits an enzyme, monoamine oxidase, in the brain—started in 1987. Monoamine oxidase works with oxygen to tear apart neurotransmitters. The neurotransmitter most involved in Parkinson's disease is dopamine, which plays an important part in movement. The idea was to determine whether the progression of Parkinson's disease could be delayed with selegiline and/or vitamin E. The results have been equivocal.[42]

Does vitamin E have potential for treatment of parkinsonism? In a meta-analysis of eighty-five parkinsonism studies, reviewers determined that vitamin E may have protectant antioxidant properties, but not enough research information with patients was available.[43]

Tardive dyskinesia is another brain condition involving abnormal movements, especially of the tongue, lips, and facial muscles. One of the causes is high doses of antipsychotic drugs given over a long period of time. Patients with tardive dyskinesia showed improvement in the symptoms in four clinical trials—double-blind and placebo-controlled—with vitamin E in dosages of up to 1,600 IUs per day.[44]

Vitamins E and A Together in Down's Syndrome and Aging

Vitamin A is necessary for keen eyesight. Through eyesight, we gain most of the information we feed our brains. A deficiency of vitamin A has also been found, at least in laboratory animals, to affect balance and cause abnormalities in taste and smell, two senses intimately involved in eating. As with vitamin E, vitamin A is an antioxidant and that may be one of its major benefits as far as the brain is concerned. The two vitamins showed potential in research concerning Down's syndrome. Formerly referred to as mongolism, Down's syndrome is a result of a genetic abnormality that produces mental retardation and usually early death. Down's syndrome patients have a tendency for their blood fats to be easily oxidized. This fat peroxidation causes progressive tissue damage.

A study from the Brain-Behavior Research Center of the University of California, San Francisco, involved twelve Down's patients and twelve non-Down's subjects. Researchers noted that the antioxidant defense system seemed overwhelmed in Down's syndrome, and that blood samples results from Down's patients demonstrated that both vitamins A and E were significantly decreased and oxidized blood fats were significantly increased. The California researchers concluded that Down's individuals have a greater than normal requirement for both vitamins

A and E to help prevent oxidative tissue damage. Could this be why Down's syndrome subjects are at risk for developing Alzheimer's disease and dementia as early as twenty or thirty years of age?

British researchers wanted to find out. They compared the blood levels of vitamin E in twelve Down's syndrome subjects with those of subjects with Alzheimer's disease. The results showed that these Down's victims did indeed have lower levels of Vitamin E than a similar group of twelve Down's subjects without Alzheimer's.[45]

The link between the low levels of the antioxidant vitamins and the rapid aging in the brains of Down's syndrome people has spurred on researchers to determine whether vitamin E and vitamin A may help protect the brains of us all, against Alzheimer's and other memory problems. In 1997, indeed, researchers at UCLA reported vitamin E can slow the progression of Alzheimer's disease.

Vitamin C and the Brain Under Stress

Another of the antioxidant vitamins, vitamin C, may also serve as a medication for the brain, particularly when it is under stress. The level of vitamin C in the brain is second only to that found in the adrenal glands.[46] The adrenal glands produce the hormones needed for fight or flight when you feel threatened. They speed the heart rate, increase the blood pressure, and generally rev up the body. These stress changes, if they occur too frequently, may cause permanent damage to the brain, heart, and other organs. This has led researchers to believe that vitamin C plays an important role in fighting stress—both emotional and physical. Smoking and drinking alcoholic beverages, for example, physically stress brain tissues because they produce free radicals, those extremely reactive, unstable, damaging molecules. Such bad habits may be made a little less harmful by using vitamin C as a nutraceutical. As the other antioxidant nutraceuticals do, vitamin C helps prevent free-radical damage.

Vitamin C may also have another way of protecting the brain. The interplay between vitamin C and amino acids, the building blocks of protein, suggests that vitamin C may play a vital role in the regulation of messages sent between the brain's nerve cells. Vitamin C has been found to be needed as a helper in the manufacture of brain neurotransmitters that act as stimulants and coordinate movements. Vitamin C also participates in the processing of glucose, blood sugar, the brain's primary food.

Multivitamins and the Brain

An ordinary multivitamin-mineral supplement was given to thirty Welsh schoolchildren (twelve- and thirteen-year-olds) who had been obtaining micronutrients from their diets at close to recommended dietary allowance levels. The study went on for eight months. Thirty of their classmates with similar diets received placebos, and thirty took no pills. The group taking the supplement had significantly increased scores on a test of nonverbal intelligence compared to both control groups. The supplement provided most vitamins in amounts well above U.S. RDA levels.[47]

Dietary deficiencies in the elderly, especially vitamins B-6 and B-12, niacin, folic acid, thiamine, and vitamin C have been well documented. Yet clinical signs of deficiency are rare. Much more common are nonspecific symptoms, such as malaise, irritability, sleepiness, loss of appetite and weight, and impairment of physical performance socially or at work. Therefore, supplemental vitamins may be needed. Most investigators feel that the benefits of multivitamin supplementation greatly outweigh any possible complications of their use.[48]

Minerals for Mood and Mind

Calcium, a fairly soft, silvery white alkaline earth metal, is the fifth most abundant element. Calcium is most often thought of as a nutrient for bones, teeth, and stomach acid, but its ingestion may also have an effect on mood.[49] Texas A & M professor Kaymar Arasteh told a meeting of the American Psychological Association that depressed patients given 1,000 milligrams of calcium gluconate plus 600 international units of vitamin D twice a day for four weeks showed significant elevation in mood compared to a control group of depressed patients who received placebos. Dr. Arasteh noted that calcium's effect on nerves in the brain and on mood is biphasic; that is, a little stimulates the nerves and elevates mood, but a lot can depress nerve activity and mood.

Calcium has long been suspected as a cause of changes in the structure and function of nerve cells and in the physiology of learning. One implication is that diets deficient in calcium severely disrupt or handicap learning.[50]

Deficiencies in iron and zinc have also been correlated with problems in cognition.

Iron was found to help the cognitive performance of mildly deficient three- to six-year-olds in Cambridge, Massachusetts. The children, after being given iron supplements, improved on three discrimination-learning tasks. It was shown that bringing their iron levels to normal had a great beneficial affect on their ability to pay attention. Again, iron should not be taken unless a physician has tested you and prescribed it.[51]

A diet deficient in zinc was found to cause memory and learning impairment in the offspring of laboratory rats fed the diets during pregnancy and suckling periods. A report in the British medical journal *Lancet* also cited zinc as a factor in the onset of genetically based senility. Foods that are high in zinc include meat, oysters, nuts, liver, and wheat germ.[52]

How Bad Does It Hurt?

Diet may not only affect how we think and behave but how we feel pain. Pain is basically a protective mechanism. The brain senses pain signals designed to make us aware that something is wrong in some area of our bodies and that action must be taken to correct it. Unfortunately, even after we are informed by our pain that something is amiss, those uncomfortable pain signals may continue to be received by our brains. Pain signals may be dampened by controlling the intake of sugar and salt.

Frank G. Lawlis, Ph.D., and his colleagues at North Texas State University's Clinical Ecology and Chronic Pain Patient Clinic, reported at the 1984 American Psychological Association results of studies involving sugar and salt. Dr. Lawlis said that when sugar enters the bloodstream at a very high rate, the pancreas produces a rush of insulin to stabilize the levels in the bloodstream and, as a result of the overproduction, the blood glucose is washed out and drops lower than before the sugar was ingested. The temporary high blood-sugar and insulin level, however, may produce a feeling of relief. Some patients perceive this stage as feeling high and happier, while others relate it to a state of increased relaxation. It does not last very long. Since the brain uses glucose in the production of endorphins, its own self-made pain killers and pleasure producers, pain symptoms and a depressed mood may appear or worsen when blood-sugar levels become unbalanced.[53]

The second food substance that may greatly affect the brain's perception of pain, the Texas researchers maintain, is sodium in the form of salt. Physiologically, sodium makes the interior of the blood vessels soggy, producing higher blood pressure. If you have an inflammation anywhere in your body or swelling, increased pressure will cause the pain to get worse. Scar tissue is also affected by the same mechanism.

Some foods, the Texans maintain, can help decrease pain. Tryptophan, an amino acid discussed in detail earlier in this chapter, is a stimulant of the brain's endorphins. Bananas, for example, have high levels of tryptophan as well as high levels of potassium, an element that when depleted causes muscle spasms. Muscle spasms, of course, can cause pain. Other foods that produce good results are almonds, melons, and grapes. The pain researchers also recommend potatoes and pastas as foods that help balance blood sugar. They appear to break down into blood sugar very slowly over the course of a day, thus helping to keep blood-sugar levels in balance. Rice cakes, popcorn, and water help a patient to feel full. Water in copious amounts is recommended because as muscles exercise, they give off lactic acid, which causes soreness. Water can help get rid of the lactic acid.

A small amount of white wine may be beneficial for pain and stress. Beer, however, can be a problem because of its high sodium levels. Highly distilled liquors such as gin, vodka, and whiskey have a disastrous effect, the Texans have found. They speculate it is because alcohol disintegrates the brain's own pain-killing system, the endorphins.

The Caffeine Charge

Caffeine, even more than alcohol, is a substance widely consumed for it behavioral effects—stimulation and abatement of drowsiness and fatigue. It quickly makes its presence felt in the brain and other organs in the body. It occurs naturally in several plant components, including the coffee bean, tea leaf, kola nut, cacao seed, and ilex leaf. The average American consumes 2 to 3 milligrams per kilogram of his or her body weight per day. One cup of coffee contains between 75 and 120 mg. Caffeine is also present in soft drinks and over-the-counter medications, including analgesics, appetite suppressants, and stimulants. If you ingest about 400 to 500 mgs. of coffee per day and show no effects from this large intake, you may have become physically dependent on caffeine.

Caffeine, which is readily absorbed, affects the central nervous system, respiratory and cardiovascular systems, smooth and skeletal muscle, gastrointestinal secretion, the rate of urine formation, and the basal metabolic rate. The brain, however, seems to be the most sensitive to caffeine. The time it takes to fall asleep is doubled in some people by a single serving of 1 to 2 milligrams of caffeine. One can see the alerting affect of caffeine in those that regularly consume it. However, in those who are *not* normally coffee drinkers, the same dose can cause irritability and nervousness. Caffeine deprivation can cause the same symptoms in regular users.

Caffeine's halflife—the time it is active—in smokers is three to four hours instead of five to six hours. The known association between increased caffeine consumption and cigarette smoking could depend, in part, on the fact that more caffeine is needed to obtain an effect on a smoker's mood.

Since caffeine produces arousal, you would expect that it increases blood flow, but a cup or two of coffee actually decreases blood flow to the brain significantly. In fact, it has been used for that purpose in treating migraines, in which the blood vessels in the brain are distended. Another paradoxical effect of coffee is that it is sometimes used to test children for hyperactivity. In many who are truly hyperactive, coffee acts to calm them down instead of stimulate them. The reasons why are not clear, but similar results have been observed with stimulant drugs.

The Brain's Appetite Center

If you have a stubborn problem with your weight, brain researchers are working on that. Investigators at Tufts and Temple universities and the National Institute of Mental Health have discovered that by giving genetically obese mice and rats naloxone, a drug that counteracts endorphins, the mice stopped overeating. The researchers conclude that their data suggests that beta-endorphin in the master gland, the pituitary, may play a role in the development of the overeating and obesity syndrome.[54]

There are other researchers working on identifying the chemicals that turn on and off the "appetite regulating center" in the hypothalamus. Many self-producing substances have been considered; among them, the neurotransmitter dopamine, the endorphins, and the fatty acids. The suspects for stimulating appetite include the neurotransmitters norepinephrine and adenosine, the hormones insulin and thyrotrophin-releasing factor, as well as an amino acid active in the brain, GABA (gamma-aminobutyric acid).

The National Institute of Child Health and Human Development (NICHD) now supports research on the relationship between nutrition and behavior to further probe the intriguing but contradictory and puzzling findings of researchers thus far. As the NICHD Guide for Researchers points out:

> Behind the expression of all ingestive behavior lies the neurophysiology and neurochemistry of hunger and satiety. Important observations on the effect of nutrient intake on levels of cerebral neurotransmitters such as serotonin and acetylcholine have been made that pave the way for studies on the influence of diet on behavior.[55]

As the mysteries of the brain and its appetite center unravel, there may prove to be easier means of controlling your appetite. In the meantime, you'll just have to use your brain to regulate what you feed it.

10

Protecting Your Brain Against Potentially Harmful Chemicals

We may think drunks at a party who stagger around and act silly are funny, but it is really no laughing matter. What has happened to them is that alcohol has affected their brains, throwing off their coordination and muddling their thinking.

Whether we were aware of it or not, every one of us has at one time or another bypassed our protective blood-brain barrier and instilled some toxin into our central nervous system. Among the many common chemicals that may affect our brains and nerves are foods, food additives, medicines, household products, and recreational substances. Volumes could be written about common chemicals in our lives that are potentially harmful to our central nervous system, and in this chapter we will try to give you a few of the more common examples.

Alcohol and the Brain

It has been known for a long time that alcohol destroys brain cells. The brains of chronic alcoholics are softer than normal. Although alcohol probably exerts widespread effects on the nervous system, the fact that human alcoholics often show severe memory disorders provides a clue that alcohol does, indeed exert a primary toxic effect on the hippocampus, a major player in memory function of the brain.[1] Current research on alcohol and the brain suggests that the symptoms alcoholics suffer are similar to those suffered by persons who have brain damage and not similar to the symptoms of normal aging.[2]

New research is explaining intoxication, tolerance, and withdrawal.

Our brains have been found to have receptors for their own self-produced opiates, the endorphins. The endorphins fit into these receptors like pegs into pegboards. These same receptors also act as depots for other opiates or psychoactive drugs we ingest. After long-term exposure to alcohol, the number of opiate receptors in the brain apparently increases.

A self-made opiate *methionine-enkephalin,* for example, has a soothing message. If it cannot bind to the appropriate receptor it cannot deliver its comfort.[3]

Although alcohol initially inhibited the endorphin's binding, the researchers found that nerve cells adapted to this blockade by increasing the number of *methionine-enkephalin* binding sites. This fits in with the common observations that chronic alcoholics and drug abusers have to keep increasing their intake of psychoactive substances to get an effect.

This is not to say that alcohol is all bad. In fact, drinking a few glasses of beer or wine each week has been found to be beneficial to the intellectual ability of a large number of elderly people. In a recent study of more than two thousand persons with an average age of seventy-four years, those who were light alcohol drinkers—fewer than four drinks per week—exhibited slightly yet consistently higher scores on tests measuring mental function than those who reported drinking ten or more drinks per week.

People who never drank alcohol or drank what was considered moderate amounts—more than four but fewer than ten drinks each week—had test results that were equal to or slightly lower than the light drinkers.[4]

Dr. Denis Evans, co-director of the Rush Alzheimer's Disease Center at Rush Presbyterian–St. Luke's Medical Center in Chicago, commented that it is questionable whether the improved mental function resulted from light alcohol intake or other factors.[5]

Food Additives and the Brain

While the testing whether additives in our food may cause cancer is imperfect, little if any testing has been done to determine if food additives may be toxic to the brain and nerves. A number of scientists believe that neurotoxins are even more of a problem in food than cancer-causing agents.[7]

The fact that some chemicals can adversely affect the nervous system is not a new concept in regulatory toxicology. In evaluating the safety of proposed food chemicals, regulators have looked for obvious pathological changes in the structure of the brain and nerves.

This view, however, does not reflect the full spectrum of adverse effects that a neurotoxin may exert on the nervous system. In humans, neurotoxins can adversely affect a broad spectrum of behavioral functions, including the ability to learn, to interact appropriately with others, and to perceive and respond to environmental stimuli. Basically these represent everyday functions that enable people to live productive lives.[8]

Excitatory Neurotoxins

As pointed out before, we use amino acids, the building blocks of proteins, to make our own neurotransmitters that send chemical messages between our brain cells. A category of these amino acids being intensively studied is the *excitatory amino acids* (EAA).

Excitotoxins are either extracted from natural sources or manufactured in the laboratory, and have biologic properties that make them useful as food additives.[9] Glutamic acid (glutamate is its salt) derives its flavor-enhancing effects from its excitatory action on sensory taste receptors. Glutamate is a neurotransmitter that transmits messages between brain nerve cells and acts as a stimulant throughout the central nervous system. Glutamate, when combined with phenylalanine, interacts with the taste receptors, resulting in the perceived sweet taste in products such as aspartame. The FDA does not place regulatory restriction on the use of glutamic acid nor does it have a program for monitoring how or in what amount glutamate is used. Although glutamate is no longer being added to baby food, as it once was, young children are exposed to large loads of it through commercially available soups and in everything from bubble gum to soda.

The excitotoxic amino acids are unique agents that interact with the central nervous system in ways that are different from other known neurotoxins.

John Olney, M.D., professor of psychiatry at Washington University in St. Louis, Missouri, has long been a critic of glutamate, especially where it may affect the brains of children. He says it is sometimes argued that glutamic acid and aspartame are safe food additives because humans have been exposed to these compounds in one form or another for many years without sustaining harm. This argument overlooks the fact that brain and retinal damage from glutamic acid or aspartame is a silent phenomenon. When infant animals are given neurotoxic doses of glutamate or aspartame, they fail to manifest overt signs of distress while nerves in the brain and eye are actually degenerating. Indeed, there are no obvious changes in the animal's appearance or behavior until it is approaching adulthood. Thus, if glutamate or aspartame damage the hypothalamus of a human infant or child, delayed sequelae such as obesity and subtle disturbances in neuroendocrine status are the types of effects to be expected, and it would not be until adolescence or perhaps early adulthood that such effects would become clearly evident.[10]

The hypothalamus is less than the size of a peanut and weighs a quarter ounce. This small area deep within the brain also oversees appetite, blood pressure, sexual behavior, emotions, and sleep, and sends orders to the pituitary gland.

Glutamate and Heart Surgery

Johns Hopkins researchers believe they have provided the first evidence that glutamate plays a role in the brain damage that occurs during certain heart surgeries because it overstimulates brain nerve cells to the point of self-destruction.[11]

A drug, called MK-801, has been given to determine if it would block glutamate from overexciting and causing brain cells to self-destruct.

Results show that dogs receiving the drug had significantly fewer brain cells die than the dogs that weren't administered the drug. The drug works by blocking glutamate receptors on the surface of brain cells which prevents glutamate molecules from attaching.

A Preservative That Is Another Excitotoxin

Cysteine-S-sulfonic acid (CSS) is another excitotoxin and is five to ten times more potent than glutamic acid. It is generated in foods because of the preservative sulfite that is added during processing. Adverse reactions to sulfites include asthma attacks, loss of consciousness, severe life-threatening anaphylactic shock, diarrhea, and nausea occurring soon after ingesting sulfiting agents.

Protection Against Toxic Excitatory Amino Acids

It is presently not clear what role excess stimulation by normally occurring excitatory amino acids might play in the cause of Alzheimer's disease. A link has been established between these neurotransmitters and Huntington's chorea, which also results in brain and nerve degeneration. It is not clear whether this degeneration is due to the over-stimulation by EAAs or whether a target population of neurons has become particularly vulnerable. If, indeed, a role for EAA in the nerve degeneration of Alzheimer's disease is demonstrated, medications that will counteract excitatory amino acids will need to be developed.[12]

The FDA has been evaluating the safety of MSG (monosodium glutamate) since 1970. While some people admittedly have adverse reactions to MSG, the FDA maintains that the additive is safe. Indeed, the European Community's Scientific Committee for Food and the Joint Expert Committee on Food Additives of the United Nations Food and Agricultural Organization and the World Health Organization have also placed MSG in the safest category of food additives.[13] It is up to you to decide for yourself about MSG's safety based on the above. Ask yourself if MSG is a necessary additive.

As for aspartame, it was determined to be safe for the food supply by the FDA. Aspartame entered the market in 1981. It is not safe for those with an intolerance to phenylalanine, one of its components. It may also not be safe in combination with glutamate, a food additive used as a flavor enhancer. The FDA has said that the only reports of problems with aspartame have been some reports of headaches. Again, ask yourself, do you really need an artificial sweetener? If you must sweeten something, a half teaspoon of sugar is only eight calories.

The Feingold Controversy

In 1975 Dr. Benjamin Feingold, a San Francisco pediatrician, published his thesis on behavioral disorders in children. He claimed dramatic success in alleviating hyperactivity by placing patients on a diet devoid of artificial food, natural salicylates, and color additives.

While many parents confirmed the merit of his recommendations, his findings remained the object of controversy among his peers. The most recent studies do not present final answers. The evidence to date seems to show that there may be a "subpopulation" of children who are sensitive to food colorings and salicylates.

However, six years after Dr. Feingold introduced his theory, it was reported by National Institutes of Health researchers that Red Dye No. 3, erythrosine, may interfere with the neurotransmitters of the brain.

There are 81,000 pounds of Red Dye No. 3 consumed a year. It was reported earlier that erythrosine may affect the thyroid. Evidence exists in studies of both animals and humans that thyroid dysfunction may evoke neurological symptoms, emotional swings, hyperactivity, and irritability.[14]

The whole subject of food allergy is a controversial one. There is even a debate over how to test for it. The effect of a food allergy on the brain is difficult to determine. There is no doubt that if you are allergic to corn, wheat, eggs, or milk, and you ingest one of your allergens, you will not feel well and may be irritable or foggy. Food allergens are usually proteins. The fact that neurotransmitters in the brain are made from proteins suggests that brain allergies may exist. Most of the allergens can still cause reactions even after they have undergone digestion.

Just how certain foods may adversely affect the transmission of nerve chemicals or affect the brain cells themselves is a fertile field for research.

Environmental Neurotoxins

There are many chemicals in our homes, yards, and offices that can potentially adversely affect our brains. Again, this is a broad subject, but below are just some of them:

Aluminum. Inefficient water treatment has been linked to an increased risk of Alzheimer's disease, according to a Canadian study. The study showed that individuals with Alzheimer's disease were 2.6 times more likely to have lived, during their last ten years of life, in areas where concentrations of aluminum in the drinking water were higher rather than in areas where there were low levels of aluminum. "High" was defined as 100 micrograms per liter or greater. Researchers estimate that 23 percent of all cases of Alzheimer's disease in Ontario during the study period may have been caused by high aluminum concentrations. The relationship between aluminum and Alzheimer's is not fully understood. Some research suggests that other chemicals in the water may alter the toxic effect of aluminum, and the concentrations of those other chemicals varies from location to location. Age itself might affect how much aluminum is absorbed by the body.

Glues, Cements, and Adhesives. Youngsters discovered the brain-muddling effects of these products. Chronic glue sniffers develop nerve damage. Some acute effects of inhalation abuse are similar to those of alcohol abuse. Most affect the brain and may cause sudden death by disrupting the rhythm of the heart.

Pesticides. Some, of course, are deadly poisons that kill quickly; others, such as those from carbamates, may do their damage more slowly. Check and heed all pesticide labels before each use and use as infrequently as possible.

DEET. An insect repellent, it is especially active against mosquitos, biting flies, gnats, chiggers, ticks, and fleas. DEET is in most repellents ranging in concentration from 7 percent to 100 percent. It is listed on the labels as N,N-diethyl-m-toluamide. Both Maximum Strength Off and Maximum Strength Cutter are 100 percent DEET. DEET is absorbed through the skin. In 1991 New York State health officials warned consumers not to use insect repellents with high levels of the chemical. DEET produced neurological problems in children such as loss of coordination and mental confusion.

Lacquer Thinner. This product may contain toluene which can be abused by inhalation and cause nerve and brain damage, hallucinations, lethargy, and coma.

Lead Compounds. Lead can enter your body in two ways: inhalation and ingestion. You can inhale lead when lead dust, mist, or fumes are present in the air you breathe. Particles of lead can be swallowed if lead gets on your hands, skin, or beard, or if it gets in your food or drinks. Other sources of lead include deposits that may be present in homes after years of use of leaded gasoline and from industrial sources like smelting. You can also generate lead dust by sanding lead-based paint or by scraping or heating lead-based paint. Once lead gets into your body, it stays there for a long time. The more lead in your body, the more likely that harm will occur. Among its toxic effects are leg cramps, muscle weakness, numbness, depression, brain damage, coma, and death. Children's brains are particularly vulnerable.

Prescription and Over-the-Counter Drugs

The subject of drugs and the brain could fill several books, as pointed out before, but there are certain drugs in common use that do cause problems in cognition. Some are well known to sometimes fog the mind, such as sedatives, sleeping pills, and tranquilizers. Others are often not recognized as having an effect on the ability to think clearly.

The following are some medications used to treat various ailments; a number of them are over-the-counter and may have the potential effect of interfering with memory.

Atropine. It is used to treat irregular heart rhythms and also in eye ointments and solutions to dilate the pupil for the treatment of eye irritations. It may inhibit acetylcholine transmission between nerves, thus potentially affecting memory.

Cimetidine. Tagamet. Introduced in 1976 for the treatment of stomach ulcers, it may cause reversible states of confusion and agitation.

Cycloserine. Seromycin. A prescription antibiotic used to treat tuberculosis,

Clomipramine Hydrochloride. Anafranil. A prescription tricyclic antidepressant to treat obsessions and compulsions.

Diclofenac Sodium. Voltaren. A prescription antiarthritis drug.

Isocarboxazid. Marplan. A prescription monoamine oxidase inhibitor used to treat depression and nerve pain, and one of the drugs that more often causes memory problems.

Eyebright. *Euphrasia officinalis.* Euphrasia. An annual herb native to Europe and western Asia and grown in the United States, it belongs to the figwort family. It has been mentioned in medical literature since the early 1300s. It had the reputation of being able to restore eyesight in the elderly, and is still used today as an eyewash for inflamed and tired eyes and to treat sinus congestion.

Steroids. Natural and synthetic steroids include cortisone, oral contraceptives, and anabolic hormones. These may cause adverse emotional symptoms if taken in excess.

Atenolol. Tenormin. Tenoretic. A prescription medication used to treat high blood pressure.

Antihistamines. Certain OTC antihistamines need to be warned that they may cause drowsiness or insomnia. Dr. Fran Gengo, associate professor of neurology and pharmacy at the State University of New York, Buffalo, tested the ability of healthy, young males to drive two to four hours after a common antihistamine had been administered.

"The change in reaction on the average went from 0.8 seconds to 2 seconds," Dr. Gengo noted, "which can mean the difference between life and death if a young child or dog runs out in front of your car."[15]

Timolol Maleate. Blocadren. Timolide. Timoptic. A prescription medication to treat high blood pressure and pressure in the eye.

Valproate. It is used to treat conditions such as seizures, migraine headaches, and bipolar disorders. Long-term use of valproate can cause symptoms similar to those of Parkinson's disease that are reversible when patients stop taking the drug.

Marijuana, *Cannabis sativa,* also known as grass, bhang, dagga, pot, hash. It is a central nervous system depressant, hallucinogen, and antivomiting drug. It is derived from the leaves and resin of the cannabis plant, and has been used medicinally for more than two thousand years. Virtually all recreational drugs impair memory and thinking, and some permanently damage the brain. Many young people, however, believe that one recreational drug—marijuana—is harmless.

Careful studies of college students have shown that marijuana does affect memory and general intellectual functioning. In one experiment reported in 1996, performed at McLean Hospital, Belmont, Massachusetts, one group of college students who were regular users of marijuana was compared with infrequent users. All subjects were abstinent from marijuana and other drugs for a minimum of nineteen hours before testing. Tests showed that heavy users displayed significantly greater impairment than light users on attention/executive functions, as evidenced particularly by greater perseverations on card sorting and reduced learning of word lists. The conclusion was that heavy marijuana use is associated with residual neuropsychological effects even after a day of supervised abstinence from the drug. However, the question remains open as to whether this impairment is due to a residue of drug in the brain, a withdrawal effect from the drug, or a frank neurotoxic effect from marijuana.[16]

Another study that indicates that marijuana may be harmful to brain function involves the effects of mothers smoking the drug during pregnancy. Researchers with the Ottawa Prenatal Prospective Study Group at Carleton University, in Canada, have been studying the effects of marijuana used during pregnancy since 1978. The mothers were primarily middle-class, low-risk women. The investigators found that the children at four years of age and older had increased behavioral problems and decreased performance on visual-perception tasks, language comprehension, sustained attention, and memory. The deficits did not begin showing up until the age of four, which the Canadian researchers concluded was consistent with the observation that marijuana exposure affects "executive functioning"—goal-directed behavior that includes planning, organized search, and impulse control.[17]

❋   ❋   ❋

Summing it up, the subject of medications, recreational drugs, and other chemicals in your environment that may be potentially harmful to your central nervous system is a tremendous one. The fewer man-made chemicals you ingest as food additives, liquor, and drugs, the less your chance of causing your brain problems. Do you really need that flavor enhancer or diet soda? Or that ulcer pill? Hopefully, if you are reading this book, you are interested in building your brain power. Therefore, you should be smart enough to chose to avoid as many neu-rotoxins as possible.

11

Chemicals for the Mind: The Search for Memory Enhancers

This book is about what you can do yourself to keep your brain fit and functioning well. There are circumstances, however, when a chemical boost may be needed. Pharmaceutical firms, government, and university researchers are hot on the trail of chemicals that may improve brain power. The quest will not only benefit an estimated two million Alzheimer's patients in the United States but will also benefit the rapidly increasing aging population with benign memory problems. Add to that children with learning disabilities and you can see why analysts are predicting a world wide market of more than a billion dollars for memory enhancers.

No one knows for certain what causes Alzheimer's, or for that matter what causes the forgetfulness that befalls most persons in middle age and later. There are a number of theories, including heredity, environmental toxins, lack of proper nutrition, and side effects of recreational and prescription drugs.

In the 1970s, it was discovered that there are chemicals secreted by the brain's nerve cells that send messages back and forth. There is no doubt that these chemical messengers, called neurotransmitters, are involved in memory and other cognitive functions. Scientists are now concentrating on pinpointing the deficits caused by garbled chemical conversations between brain cells.

Acetylcholine—The Memory Messenger

As we age, ability to transfer information from one cell to another or to a target organ is markedly reduced in everyone, but to a greater degree in some people than in others. This is due in part, scientists believe, to the amount of the neurotransmitter acetylcholine in the cell, and in part to the ability to use what is there. Acetylcholine is believed to be vital to memory.

Recall that old belief that fish is brain food? There may be some truth to it because fish contains high levels of choline, as do meat and eggs. Choline is taken from the food in the digestive tract by the blood and carried to the brain, where it is turned into acetylcholine.

The discovery that acetylcholine declines in Alzheimer's disease led naturally to the hypothesis that replacing acetylcholine could stop the disease. Since that finding, many scientists have looked for compounds that can either increase the levels of acetylcholine, replace it, or slow its breakdown. This search has taken them into a broad territory that includes the cells that use acetylcholine and the enzymes and other proteins that take part in its manufacture or activity—a grouping known as the *cholinergic system.*

One of the most persistent findings is that the activity of an enzyme—choline acetyltransferase (CAT)—is reduced in the aged human brain and markedly diminished in the brains of Alzheimer's patients. CAT is an enzyme used by our brains to produce acetylcholine. Interestingly, it has been discovered that stress depresses CAT levels. That helps explain why we have difficulty remembering something when we are under stress.

The discovery of acetylcholine deficits in Alzheimer's disease also raised hope that choline and lecithin, if added to the diet, could help in treating memory problems. The body uses these nutrients to synthesize acetylcholine. Trials with the two substances have been disappointing so far.

A member of the cholinergic system is another enzyme, *acetylcholinesterase* (often referred to simply as cholinesterase), the enzyme that breaks down acetylcholine after it crosses the synapse. Many of the experimental Alzheimer's drugs developed to date are cholinesterase inhibitors; that is, they are designed to suppress cholinesterase so that acetylcholine will not be broken down as quickly.

One such cholinesterase inhibitor is THA or tetrahydroaminoacridine. Under the name tacrine (Cognex) it is approved by the Food and Drug Administration to slow down the loss of cognitive ability in Alzheimer's disease. THA has helped some patients, but its impact on the disease in general has proved disappointing. However, other cholinesterase inhibitors that may be more effective are entering the market.

Medicines Used for Other Purposes That May Help the Brain

By serendipity, physicians have found that certain medications used for other purposes may have a beneficial effect on the brain.

The Anti-Inflammatories

There is growing acceptance of the idea that Alzheimer's disease may be a chronic inflammatory disorder similar to arthritis and that non-steroidal anti-inflammatory drugs (NSAIDs) may have certain beneficial effects in slowing Alzheimer's. Among the NSAIDs are the familiar aspirin, ibuprofen, and naproxen. One Canadian researcher said that twelve epidemiological studies have been published showing that patients taking anti-inflammatory medication have substantially lower prevalence of Alzheimer's disease and that in one study the anti-inflammatory drug, indomethacin, appeared to "arrest progression of the disease."[1]

In a recent study of twins, one member of each pair had Alzheimer's and the other did not. Many of the twins who did not have the disease had one thing in common: They took anti-inflammatory drugs for arthritis. A clinical trial is now testing whether the anti-inflammatory drugs can slow the progress of the disease in its early stages.

Estrogen and the Brain

In two major studies, one in the Netherlands and one in California involving hundreds of women, results did show that women who took estrogen after menopause had lower rates of Alzheimer's disease, and when they did develop the condition, it was delayed when compared to women who had never taken the therapy.[2]

Just how estrogen works in the brain remains obscure, though research by Bruce McEwen, Ph.D., at Rockefeller University, in New York City has shown that the hormone increases the number of connections between nerve cells in the hippocampus, a region that helps govern memory. Estrogen also increases the production of acetyl-choline, a brain chemical that is abnormally low in Alzheimer's patients.

Researchers have found that the cholinergic neurons of the brain have numerous estrogen receptors, and they occur on the same nerve cells that have receptors for nerve growth factor (NGF). Estrogen injected in rats' brains strongly affects nerve cells in the cerebral cortex and the hippocampus—regions of the brain affected by Alzheimer's disease. These pieces of evidence have given rise to the theory that nerve growth factor and estrogen interact in some way to protect cells involved in memory from degenerating.

Frank Bolino, M.D., of the National Institute on Aging, Bethesda, Maryland, who oversees grants for the study of menopause, says that until fairly recently, it was believed that it was strictly the ovary that caused women to go through menopause.

"We now know that the hypothalamus and the pituitary play a part in menopause and when we better understand why menopause occurs, then we will know more about its effect on bone loss, cardiovascular problems, and perhaps Alzheimer's," he says.[3]

Geriatrician Dr. Howard Fillit, a professor at Mt. Sinai Medical Center in New York City, says estrogen also has an effect on inflammation and blood vessels and new research is showing that inflammation may play a large part in the development of brain deterioration such as that seen in Alzheimer's and multiple vascular dementia.[4] Dr. Fillit also points out that estrogen can:

• modulate neurotransmitter systems (messages sent between brain cells)
• improve blood flow
• alter IL-2, a substance released by cells associated with inflammation

Both men and women have estrogen receptors throughout the brain, including some areas affected by Alzheimer's.[5]

If estrogen can prevent or delay the onset of Alzheimer's, can it also treat it? Clinical trials of estrogen as a treatment in early-stage Alzheimer's disease are underway.

Neil Buckholtz, M.D., of the National Institute on Aging, said that the findings thus far about estrogen may be the most promising advance ever made toward the prevention of Alzheimer's.

It is much too early, of course, to tell whether taking estrogen does reduce the risk of Alzheimer's disease. And since estrogen replacement therapy following menopause is not recommended for all women, scientists have urged caution in interpreting the findings to date. Men may be at a lower risk for dementia because of an enzyme called aromatase, which converts testosterone to estrogen in the brain.

Testosterone and the Brain

It has long been reported that the increases in testosterone, the major male hormone, can make men aggressive and quick to anger; a decrease in testosterone causes a decline in interest in sex and a vaguely diminished sense of well-being. The hormone's relationship to Alzheimer's has not been studied as much as estrogen's, but there are some early results that show that it may have a similar beneficial effect on the brain.

Johns Hopkins scientists reported their findings on testosterone-replacement therapy for older men. Results of their study, funded by the National Institutes of Health, were presented June 14, 1996, at the International Congress of Endocrinology's annual meeting in San Francisco. Ten men with low testosterone underwent word, memory, coordination, and other learning tests while on and off testosterone treatment. The results showed that when receiving testosterone, they had improved visual and spatial skills and a better "mental grasp of objects"—fitting building blocks into the correct spaces, identifying pictures, and remembering shapes, patterns, and locations. When not receiving testosterone, the men showed improved verbal fluency and verbal memory—making up sentences, defining words, and recalling words from a test.

"This is an interesting, early finding, and it highlights the importance of studying the effects of sex hormones on brain function," says Adrian Dobs, M.D., lead author on the study and an associate professor of medicine at Johns Hopkins.

Lower the Pressure

One of the best protections against loss of cognitive function is avoiding high blood pressure in middle age. A study of more than 3,700 Japanese American men showed that the risk of suffering serious brain dysfunction increased by 9 percent with each 10 point increase is systolic blood pressure at midlife. The systolic is the more important blood number because it measures the pressure when the heart is contracting. Lenore J. Launer, Ph.D., of the National Institute of Public Health,

Erasmus University Medical School in the Netherlands, who conducted the study, said that at the end of the investigation, when the men were an average of seventy-eight years old, they underwent cognitive function testing to measure their attention span, concentration, and memory.[6]

Hardening of the arteries in the brain, changes in its blood flow, or other physical changes in the brain may explain why high systolic blood pressure worsens mental function. So, if you can't control your blood pressure with loss of weight, exercise, and proper diet, there are high blood pressure medications that can protect your brain. Some of these medications, however, as pointed out in chapter 10 can, themselves, interfere with your thinking. If you suspect you have such side effects, check with your physician.

Insulin and Alzheimer's

The brain's main fuel is glucose—blood sugar. Can diabetes and Alzheimer's have something in common? Suzanne Craft, Ph.D., associate professor of psychology at Washington University in St. Louis, Missouri, believes they do. She has shown that infusing insulin in Alzheimer's patients improves their memory. The Washington University professor noted that one of the primary areas of brain degeneration among Alzheimer's patients is in the hippocampus, which plays an important role in memory function. She notes that there are dense concentrations of insulin receptors in certain regions of the hippocampus. Although it is known that for patients with Alzheimer's, the brain's use of glucose decreases over the course of the disease, the cause of this reduction has not been identified. Craft's findings suggest a link between the brain's ability to use insulin to regulate glucose and the progression of Alzheimer's disease.[7]

Vitamin B-12 by Injection

This vitamin helps form red blood cells and maintains a healthy nervous system. Deficiency symptoms include anemia, brain damage, and nervousness. More than one in five older Americans may need to take vitamin B-12 to prevent neurological disorders, according to a Tufts University study to prevent neurological disorders and senility. These people no longer secrete enough stomach acid to absorb the vitamin from foods. The condition, known as atrophic gastritis, affects at least 20 percent of people over the age of sixty.

Acetyl-L-Carnitine

Carnitine, a natural body substance, is essential for fatty acid oxidation and energy production. It is used in the treatment of a deficiency disease in which the brain and heart muscles are affected. Carnitine is sold in both prescription and over-the-counter forms. In the latter it is used as a dietary supplement, especially for persons with kidney disease. Acetyl-L-carnitine, a synthetic version, is being tested to slow Alzheimer's by reducing the production of free radicals that are side-products of metabolism and that damage cells. Acetyl-L-carnitine also may provide important building blocks for the brain's production of its own memory drug, acetylcholine.[8]

Do Not Deposit

Alzheimer's disease is characterized by the deposits of a protein called beta amyloid. Beta amyloid, dense deposits forming the core of tangled nerve plaques in the brain, has long been suspected of being a cause of Alzheimer's disease. It cannot be the whole story, however, because these beta-amyloid deposits are found in the brains of some older persons who do not have the disease. This residue is believed to foul up the machinery of the brain by forming plaques with tangles of nerve tissue.

The inhibition of amyloid formation has been proposed as a target for slowing the progression of Alzheimer's. The Schering and Cehpalon corporations are collaborating in the design of protease inhibitors—the same drugs that have made such therapeutic progress in the treatment of AIDS—for preventing creation of amyloid plaques.

Calcium Channel Blockers

The theory that a rise in calcium levels in neurons is the final step in the biochemical pathway leading to Alzheimer's disease has raised more treatment possibilities. Calcium channel blockers, which are widely used as a blood pressure medication, might keep this final step from taking place and thus prevent or help slow down the disease. Calcium enters and exits nerve cells through several kinds of channels, so finding the right channel and channel blocker may be a complex task. Currently, one drug company is testing a channel blocker in Alzheimer's patients and other calcium regulators are being considered for trials.

The Wake-Up Drug

Naloxone is used by anesthetists to waken patients after they have had surgery. Naloxone, which is also marketed for the treatment of drug overdoses, seems to have possibilities for the treatment of Alzheimer's.

The Search for New Drugs Is in Your Head

Like the blue bird of happiness in the backyard, pharmaceuticals that protect and improve memory may be manufactured by the brain itself. Once these chemicals can be identified, isolated, and imitated in the laboratory, the means of treating Alzheimer's, the benign but annoying memory deficits of aging, and even learning problems in children may be possible.

Nerve growth factor, for example, is believed to maintain and repair our nerves. Recent evidence, however, has shown high levels of NGF to be present in a variety of fluids after inflammatory and autoimmune responses, suggesting that NGF plays a part in immune reactions and stress.

In experiments, with young, brain-injured rats, untreated injured brain cells atrophied and died. But injured NGF-treated cells lived and sprouted new extensions. NGF seems to reverse atrophy of nerve cells in the brains of aging rats. Furthermore, it has been demonstrated that old rats with memory impairment show behavioral improvement after treatment with NGF. Similar findings have also been reported in monkeys.[9]

Researchers at Johns Hopkins have been studying the effects of NGF in rats. Dr. A. L. Markowska and colleagues point out that it is well documented that NGF ameliorates age-related deficits in certain types of memory in rats.

Human NGF was infused over a period of two and four weeks into the brains of old rats. It showed no results after two weeks but produced memory power as efficient as that of young mice after four weeks.[10]

Over-the-Counter Brain Boosters?

There are chemicals that stimulate your brain for which you do not need a prescription. The most widely used brain stimulant is caffeine. A stimulant drug that occurs in coffee, tea, and cola, it is considered the most commonly consumed drug in the United States. Caffeine is added to many analgesic medications and is used to treat breathing problems in newborns. It may be helpful in very low doses, such as a single cup of coffee, but may impair performance in high doses.

Ginkgo

Have you purchased any ginkgo balboa yet? Ginkgo is among the most popular prescription drugs in Europe. In the United States, it is sold over-the-counter as a food.

What is ginkgo? The leaves and nuts of the *Ginkgo biloba* tree— also called the Maidenhair tree—are used in ancient Chinese remedies. The ginkgo is supposedly the oldest living tree, having survived some 200 million years. It is said to be the only tree that survived the effects of atomic radiation in Hiroshima, Japan.

Ginkgo has been reported to improve circulation and mental functioning, to stop ringing in the ears, and to relieve symptoms of Alzheimer's disease, coldness, emotional depression, Raynaud's disease (a circulatory problem), arthritic disease, hardening of the arteries, dizziness, and anxiety. In recent animal studies at the University of Illinois, ginkgo protected the brains of rats to a significant degree when a toxic compound that induces oxygen damage and brain swelling was given. One explanation of its therapeutic effects is that it dilates the tiniest blood vessels in the brain, increasing blood flow and hence oxygen.[11] Excessive use can cause itching and gastrointestinal upset. In rare instances, excessive doses can induce shortness of breath and convulsions.[12]

The Chinese Secret

Scientists and pharmaceutical firms are excited about another ancient remedy, a tea, Oian Ceng Ta, brewed by elderly Chinese from the leaves of *Huperzia Serrata,* (Club Moss) to improve memory. In the 1980s, scientists at the Shanghai Institute of Materia Medica and the Zhejiang Academy of Medical Sciences isolated the active components in Huperzine (Hup A) and found that it was a remarkably potent inhibitor of acetylcholinesterase. Acetylcholinesterase, as pointed out earlier, breaks down acetylcholine, a chemical in the brain that is vital for memory function. The Chinese have reported that Hup A is effective in treating patients with memory impairment, myasthenia gravis, and multi-infarct dementia (small clots that cause mental deterioration).[13]

12

Stop Stress from Short-Circuiting Your Brain

Sigmund Freud, the pioneer psychoanalyst, made us realize the mind could paralyze the body: that emotional anguish could have a terrible effect on our flesh.

Hans Selye, M.D., the director of the University of Montreal's Institute of Experimental Medicine and the father of the "stress theory," told us that stress—both physical and emotional—could have an adverse effect on our health and actually injure organs.

Now new high-technology studies of the human brain show stress can shrink a crucial part of it. In a review article titled "Why Stress Is Bad for Your Brain" in the the journal *Science*, Professor Robert Sapolsky of Stanford University said the work of several research groups shows links between long-term stressful life experiences, long-term exposure to hormones produced during stress, and shrinking of the part of the brain involved in some types of memory and learning.[1]

Researchers can make clear images of specific parts of the brain. In his article Professor Sapolsky summarizes what has been found so far as scientists use high-resolution magnetic resonance imaging (MRI) to obtain views of the hippocampus, the sea-horse shaped area involved in stress responses.

The hippocampus is also the region of the brain responsible for implicit, declarative memory—for knowing a fact like an address or the name of a friend, and knowing that one knows it. Its neurons are rich in glucocorticoid receptors. Glucocorticoid hormones are emitted into your blood stream by your adrenal gland when you are under stress to raise your blood sugar and give you added energy. In animal studies, it has been shown that the hippocampus is the region where stress hormones can damage neurons.

Because depression can raise the levels of glucocorticoids in the blood, Dr. Yvette Sheline and her colleagues at Washington University, St. Louis, Missouri, compared the hippocampi of people who had recovered from long-term, major depression with controls matched to them by age, education, gender, and height. They found that people with a history of depression had smaller hippocampi—averaging as much as 15 percent smaller in volume.

Drs. Tamara Gurvits and Roger Pitman of Harvard found that this region of the brain was 26 percent smaller in Vietnam veterans with post-traumatic stress disorder than in combat veterans without stress disorder. Dr. Douglas Bremner of Yale found a 12 percent atrophy in the left hippocampus of adults who suffered from post-traumatic stress disorder because of childhood sexual abuse.

While there is yet much to learn about this process, there seems to be little doubt that stress can kill brain cells. One of the most graphic examples of the physical effects of stress on the brain was reported by Danish doctors. They took CAT scans of young men between twenty-four and thirty-nine years of age who had been victims of political torture. The doctors found that the young men had premature "aging of their brains." All of the men had been healthy and intelligent before being tortured, but their brains were seen on the X-rays to be atrophied. During examinations, the men's ability to concentrate and their memories were impaired. The former prisoners suffered headaches, anxiety, depression, numbness, sleep disturbances, and sexual dysfunction.[2]

The Danish doctors said that tortured men had symptoms similar to the social and mental complications experienced by victims of concentration camps during World War II. The young men's brains probably had been permanently damaged by stress chemicals secreted when they were tortured.

Torture and experience in concentration camps are extreme forms of stress. But in studies by researchers with the support of the National Institute on Aging, it has been found that if a person does not cope well with everyday stresses, physical problems that shorten life can also result.

National Institute On Aging grantee Richard S. Lazarus, working at the University of California at Berkeley, assessed the responses of one hundred men and women, forty-five to sixty-four years of age, to daily

stresses as well as major life events.[3] Subjects kept a daily log and responded to questionnaires and interviews about sources of stress—
from minor annoyances to major problems and how they felt—happy,
guilty, or fearful for example.

Dr. Lazarus found that the frequency of the irritations of everyday life—such as traffic jams or broken appointments or having to
rush—as well as the uplifts, were more powerful predictors of psychological and physical health and morale then were major life events.

But, as many others have pointed out, *it is not what you meet in
daily life so much as how you meet it that really counts.* Lazarus found
that a subject's view of a problem had an important impact on coping.
Participants who felt they could change a situation tended to use
problem-solving techniques rather than emotional responses such as
seeking sympathy, feeling bad, or blaming themselves. In other words,
they used their heads to solve their problems instead of fretting about
them.

Researchers at Duke University found that reactions to mental
stress may be a much better indicator of who will suffer heart problems
than reactions to physical stress, like running on a treadmill. The study
found that mental stress tests were better at predicting future heart
problems than physical testing alone. The study of 126 people for five
years showed that 27 percent of the patients who responded adversely
to mental stress testing, which could include public speaking or solving complex mathematical problems on a tight deadline, suffered a
heart attack. Only 12 percent of those who failed the test were free of
heart trouble, the study found.[4]

Duke psychologist Dr. James Blumenthal, said, "By potentially reducing the abnormal responses to mental stress you might reduce the
risk for future cardiac events."

How you cope, therefore, affects how old your brain is physiologically. Furthermore, there is growing scientific conjecture that brain
aging may act as a "pacemaker" for other forms of aging, particularly
through the deregulation of hormones that act on the central nervous
system.

While these studies do not absolutely prove that stress shrinks the
brain, it is known that in Cushing's syndrome, caused by a tumor that
stimulates the adrenal glands to produce large amounts of stress hormones, the patients' hippocampi show the same sort of shrinkage.

The good news is that Sapolsky found in rats short-term exposure
to stress hormones causes neurons to shrink, but they rebound when

levels of the hormones return to normal. Long-term exposure causes irreversible damage.

Your Brain-Body Connection

Your brain and your body converse with electrochemical signals. There is a sensitive "biofeedback" between them. Your brain says one thing and your body responds. Your body makes a suggestion and your brain answers.

Neuroscientists are rapidly becoming able to decode these conversations. They already know a great deal about how illness, injury, inactivity, and emotional upsets may garble the messages. They are confirming what witch doctors have known all along: Thoughts emanating from your brain can cure or kill your body.

Your brain has a built-in chemical alarm system that was identified by Dr. Selye. When you perceive danger in the environment, your brain sends signals to ready your body to "fight or flee." The key word is *perceives*, because something may be stressful to you that may not bother someone else and vice versa.

Stress, which can be either threatening or pleasurable, causes a reported one thousand chemical and physical changes in your brain and body.[5] For example, stress stimulates the production of hormones, those powerful substances manufactured by endocrine glands to orchestrate body functions. Blood levels of the hormones epinephrine (adrenaline), norepinephrine, cortisol, growth hormone, and glucagon, for example, rise under stress. These endocrine products speed metabolism. Other hormones that increase under stress include antidiuretic hormone (ADH), which enhances water reabsorption into the blood stream; aldosterone, which increases salt retention by the body, and thus water retention; oxytocin, which induces muscle contractions; and renin and angiotensin, which play a role in blood pressure elevation.

On the other hand, certain hormones are suppressed during stress, including insulin, needed to regulate blood sugar; thyroid hormone, which regulates metabolism; and the male sex hormone testosterone. In the female, sex hormones fall out of synchrony under stress and can cause the menstrual cycle to become irregular or absent.

In 1996 British doctors reported what they termed *Psychosocial Short Stature.* They found that children who failed to grow despite the fact there was no organic pathology came from stressful homes. The growth hormone from their pituitary gland behind the nose at the base of the brain was found to be deficient. When the children were removed from their homes, their pituitary glands spontaneously began to put out a sufficient supply of the hormone and the children grew normally.[6]

All of the hormones mentioned above normally regulate specific physiological functions that help maintain the body in exquisite balance. When the body is stressed for short periods of time, the effects of stress hormones in a healthy person may be transient. However, when the stress response is prolonged, then the persistent elevation of some hormones and suppression of others can have deleterious effects on the body, including increased blood levels of cholesterol and blood-clotting factors and an increase in blood pressure.

Scientific studies have concluded that from 75 to 90 percent of the ills that afflict us are due to stress. For example, young men—aged twenty-eight to thirty-five—working on the man-to-the moon project at the Kennedy Space Center in the 1960s had a 50 percent higher incidence of cardiovascular disorders and sudden death than did age- and sex-matched controls. The frenzied pace, national attention, and manpower cuts produced high stress and frustration levels. More and more evidence is being gathered to prove that stress depresses the body's defense system. A team at Mt. Sinai Medical Center in New York City, for instance, found that the immune function in husbands of terminally ill breast-cancer patients was affected, and susceptibility to disease was at the height three months after the wives died. Most of the widowers' immune systems returned to prebereavement levels by six months.[7]

Stress can even effect the unborn. The hippocampus has the most binding sites for stress hormones in the brain. Researchers now theorize that when a pregnant woman is exposed to environmental stress, the raised levels of stress hormones in her blood may permanently alter her fetus's hippocampus and thus affect her offspring's response to stress in adulthood. This has been proven to be true in rats whose mothers were stressed during pregnancy.[8]

Stress may prematurely age the adult brain. National Institute on Aging grantee Philip Landfield of the Bowman Gray School of Medicine points out that the brain deterioration seen in older people and that seen in younger people with Cushing's syndrome, a rapid and premature form of aging associated with high levels of adrenal (stress) hormones, are quite similar. Over the years, Dr. Landfield has found that the blood levels of adrenal hormones in experimental animals correlate significantly with the degree of age-related changes in the brain.[9]

This seems quite logical when you consider that the brain structures that receive and send "emotional" information are called, collectively, the limbic system. One portion about the size of a half dollar, the amygdala, is involved in rage, anger, and fear behaviors. The hippocampus beside it, as noted, is the target area of the adrenal gland's stress hormones that prepare the body for fight or flight. The continuous bombardment of stress hormones on the brain appears to kill off some of the stress-hormone receptors in the hippocampus.[10] As a result, researchers believe, the hippocampus's ability to shut off the system weakens. Thus, through a feedback circuit, the brain's limbic system, the control center of emotions, gradually destroys itself.

The Stress of Pain and the Brain

Pain is a common and powerful stress as the victims of torture mentioned before graphically illustrated. Just as fear prepares us to fight or flee, pain signals our brains that something is damaging our bodies. The nerve endings that respond to pain are nociceptors—from the Greek *noci*, meaning "noxious." These nociceptors are present in the skin, in sheath tissue surrounding muscles, in internal organs, and in the membranes around the bone and around the cornea of the eye.

There are two levels of response. The first takes place almost as a reflex. You touch your toe to bath water that is too hot and you withdraw it instantly. Then there are aches and longer-lasting pains. In the first instance, the swift pain message is carried by myelinated (coated), thin fibers. In the second instance, unmyelinated, slow-conducting fibers produce a diffuse, nagging pain.

The fibers of the *fast pathway* make direct connections with the thalamus, where they are next to the fibers that project to motor and sensory areas of the higher brain, the cortex. This allows you to discriminate exactly where the injury is, how serious the damage, and how long it has been going on.

The fibers of the *slow pathway* project to many areas of the brain, including the hypothalamus and the thalamus and the "emotional" areas of the limbic system. It is believed that the fast system gets us out of danger quickly and that the slow system reminds us to take it easy, we have an injury.

There is also a neurotransmitter that is the subject of a great deal of research today, substance P, a nerve chemical that rapidly builds up after injury. When present in abundance at one segment of the spinal cord, the pain impulses arriving at that segment are enhanced and augmented in their transmission toward the brain. Substance P has also been found in the brain cells, so it probably has functions beside the transmission of pain impulses.

Neuroimmunologist Donald G. Payan, M.D., assistant professor of medicine at the University of California, San Francisco, reported at an American Association for the Advancement of Science meeting that he has traced radioactive-labeled substance P. He has found that it binds most readily with "Helper T Cells," a type of white blood cell that stimulates the body's immune system. He and other researchers believe substance P may be involved in autoimmune diseases such as arthritis and allergies where the body's defenses are overactive and injure tissue.[11]

The endorphins, as mentioned many times in this book, are our own self-produced neurotransmitters that counteract pain and other stress once we have recognized the danger. If there were no such system, we would be unable to think to save ourselves or to do something about the cause of pain. The endorphin-producing brain cells are logically concentrated in the limbic system, that part of the brain closely linked with strong emotion. This apparent connection between natural pain-relieving substances and the brain's emotional centers led researchers to wonder if it could explain placebo effect. (The term *placebo* from the Latin "I shall please" signifies a medically inert substance, such as a sugar pill or a saline injection, that is given to patients who have been deluded into thinking they are receiving a potent medicine.)

Patients undergoing the extraction of wisdom teeth, a painful process, volunteered for a test of the placebo effect. Scientists administered morphine post-operatively to one group and injected saline into another group. Thirty-three and a third percent of those receiving the inert saline injection had a dramatic reduction in pain. Then scientists administered doses of a drug, naloxone, which is known to interfere with the body's production of endorphins. Those in whom the placebo injection had relieved their pain immediately developed shooting pains. This proved, as far as the researchers were concerned, that those volunteers given saline shots and who had relief of pain received the benefit of their own increased endorphin activity. It also became clear that the placebo effect, far from being a mind-over-matter mystery, has a definite basis in matter—the chemicals of the brain.

And like morphine, the body's own morphinelike chemicals may cause an addiction. Bessel A. Van derKilk, M.D., professor of psychiatry at Harvard Medical School, and other researchers have shown that prolonged stress, like the administration of opiates, activates the opiate receptors in animal brains. When stressed animals received naloxone, which counteracts opiates, or are removed from stress, they develop opiate-withdrawal symptoms. This has led to the conclusion that chronically stressed animals may become physically dependent on self-made opioids that are released by the brain to counteract pain and other stresses.[12]

Edgar Wilson, M.D., and Carol Schneider, Ph.D., of the University of Colorado, at a meeting of the Biofeedback Society of America suggested that one cause of chronic pain may be due to the brain being bombarded by painful sensory inputs from one area of the body over a prolonged period of time. It then tends to become more and more sensitive to those inputs because its self-made opioid supply may become depleted.[13]

Another cause of chronic pain, according to Drs. Wilson and Schneider, may be that the cerebellum, which controls movement, develops an irregular movement pattern because the affected muscles are out of synchronicity. They point out that each of us has a holding side of our bodies and a pivot side—usually the dominant side of the brain determines this. If you are right-handed, you are most likely to stand on your right foot when talking and pivot on your left side when you move.

The difference between chronic-pain patients and people who routinely run two or three miles a day, they found, was a marked difference in movement pattern. The pain patients tended to shuffle along, with their shoulders thrust forward, their heads down, their toes turning slightly inward; the general orientation of body movement was from side to side. Runners, instead, had a more vertical orientation of movement. Their shoulders were held back, as well as their heads. The runners, however, leaned into their walks rather than resisting the next step.

The Colorado researchers said that you can prevent painful "trigger points" in your muscles by working on the symmetry of your movement and on improving your posture:

• Check your movement symmetry by looking at a pair of your old tennis shoes or Oxfords. Are the bottom of the shoes worn in a symmetrical pattern or is there a distinct difference between the left and right shoe?

• Watch a slowed-down home movie or videotape of your movements and try to observe the areas of your body that you hold back as you move.

In addition to imbalances in movement, the Colorado researchers cited the neurotransmitter serotonin as a possible contributor to chronic pain. Serotonin, which is believed to inhibit reflex action, may be depleted by spasms.

How can pain messages to the brain be interrupted?

We know that we can do it surgically by making tiny lesions with very fine instruments in the spinal cord or in the front of the brain.[14] This is a mechanical method that "cuts" the communication of even the most agonizing pain.

We can also do it chemically, but not as effectively, with pharmaceutical pain killers. However, as scientists learn more and more about the brain's own neurotransmitters, more effective pain suppressants will be available. What has been learned thus far seems to explain why one of the most ancient pain-control methods works—counterirritation. Acupuncture, for example, more than two thousand years old, involves the twirling of needles in tissues to produce a deep, aching sensation. Cupping, in which a hot cup is placed on the skin, causes painful bruises and is almost as old as acupuncture. The Vietnamese rub a coin against the skin to treat pain. Athletic trainers today use ice to treat the injuries of athletes. The ice causes pain and so does electrical stimulation. Transcutaneous (through the skin) stimulators are increasingly popular electronic devices that are employed to treat all sorts of pain, from mild to severe. Pain inhibits pain, most likely by one pain perception interfering with the perception of another and affecting the release of neurotransmitters.

How much control do we have over our own neurotransmitters? We have potentially a great deal, but just as we don't use our full capacity to learn and perform, we don't use our full powers to modulate the chemical conversations that go on between our brains and our bodies.

Stress and Heart and Brain Conversations

The conversation between heart and brain during stress is probably most obvious. Remember how you felt when someone to whom you were very attracted sexually walked into the room, or when you sat in the dentist's chair awaiting the drilling? Your heart beat faster than usual. According to husband-and-wife research team John and Beatrice Lacey, at the Fels Research Institute, Yellow Springs, Ohio, not only is your heart rate sensitive to what your eyes see, but your eyes and brain respond as if controlled by the internal workings of your heart. There is a feedback. The Laceys maintain that the brain and heart/blood pressure form a feedback system with the brain continuously instructing the heart and the heart exhorting the brain. Under stressful conditions when it may be necessary to fight or flee, the heart accelerates, the blood pressure rises, and the body is prepared to react physically. On the other hand, when the brain is concentrating on an environmental or intellectual problem, the heart rate slows down.

In their experiments, the Laceys found that increases in heart rate and blood pressure interfere with attention to external environmental events, while decreases "tune in" the external world more sharply.[15]

Brain, Heart, and Personality

So your heart affects your brain's ability to concentrate while your brain affects the ability of your heart to beat regularly.

In the 1970s, two San Francisco cardiologists, Ray Rosenman, M.D., and Meyer Friedman, M.D., described the personality type that was most prone to cardiovascular disease. People who were hard driving, competitive, and impatient were labeled Type A and said to be at greater risk than the more placid, labeled Type B.

In a study in the 1980s, the findings of Rosenman and Meyer held true, even in schoolboys. The blood pressure and heart rate of a group of youngsters were monitored as they played video games. The boys were then interviewed and their personality characteristics identified. Results of the study showed that the boys classified as Type A in interviews had a rise in blood pressure and heart rate greater than did those classified as Type B.

Dr. Karen A. Matthews, who directed the study, pointed out that normally blood pressure and heart rate increase during any task performance. But those increases found in Type A boys were greater than in Type Bs, and the nature of their blood pressure changes indicates more involvement than the usual physiologic response.

The more placid boys' blood pressures went up an average of 10 millimeters of mercury while the more competitive type had a 12 millimeter rise. Heartbeats for the competitive increased eight beats per minute while the Type Bs had a increase of only three per minute.[16]

Research such as the investigation with the boys has led to the conclusion that part of your physical reaction to stress is genetic. Your brain perceives the environment and sends alerting chemical signals to your body with equipment inherited from your mother or father. Some people's nervous systems are more "sensitive" and react more strongly than others. However, you also learn through experience, just like Pavlov's dog, to react to certain situations with alarm. The big question is, how much control can you gain over your stress reactions, despite heredity and learning?

Start with New Awareness

All of the above tells you that stress can be bad for your brain. You know it, but what can you do about it. The first thing to do is to be aware that you are under stress. In today's fast-paced world, you may be so busy that you fail to recognize the signs. Here are some of them:

• Stop. Are your shoulders and neck tense? If so, you probably are.

• Do you bite your nails, pull on your hair, and/or tap your feet or fingers?

• Are you addicted to food, candy, alcohol, coffee, or other stimulants or downers?

• Do you have trouble falling asleep and/or wake up in the morning tired?

• Do you suffer frequent headaches, neckaches, backaches, or high blood pressure?

• Are you accident prone?

• Do you make a lot of mistakes?

• Are you frequently short-tempered?

All of the above are frequent signs of stress and signals that you have to practice relaxing.

Methods of Relaxation and Control

You can even gain control of those functions that Western medical textbooks describe as involuntary, such as your digestion and heartbeat. Even your state of consciousness can be affected by how you voluntarily use your brain.

Eastern religious practitioners have known this all along. The yogis, for example, have emphasized the study and expansion of consciousness. They maintain that there is a positive realization of the body's capacities for sensory experience, for self-regulating of many body functions, and for avoiding the "aging" stresses in daily living. The yogis perform movements that consciously exercise the body and the mind together and have proven that humans can have amazing control over their own heartbeats and respirations.

Biofeedback

Western researchers today have applied learning and motivation to physiological functions formerly labeled involuntary and have constructed a scientific basis for what is now called biofeedback. The technique is based upon the learning principle that a desired response is learned when received information (feedback) indicates that a specific thought or action has produced the desired response.

You use a form of biofeedback all the time. The simple act of maintaining your balance involves complex reflexes elicited by feedback from your eyes, your inner ear, and your sense organs in muscles and joints. As you read this, tilt as far as you can off the side of the chair. Did you feel your neck and head trying to right your body? Information that you tilted slightly to one side elicited your reflexes to correct that tilt.

When these feedback mechanisms are disrupted, as in sea sickness or zero gravity in space, nausea and other symptoms of motion sickness are often elicited. Yet people can be trained to control such symptoms by the use of biofeedback devices combined with relaxing imagery. The air force has found that such training can restore to flying status aircrew who might otherwise be grounded because of air sickness.

At New Jersey Neurological Institute we use biofeedback to treat pregnant women with migraine headaches. This avoids potential adverse effects from medications for the mother or the fetus. We also use biofeedback to reduce high blood pressure. It can supplement medication and reduces the quantity needed.

The primary difference between biofeedback and other self-regulation therapies is the use of electronic instrumentation that records and feeds back to you information about your body functions that you have never had before. The feedback may be in the form of a computerized video display or a simple light or tone that fluctuates along with the biological signal being monitored. With the use of such devices, and with the guidance of a biofeedback therapist, most people can easily learn to bring under voluntary control such phenomena as muscle tension and blood flow to the limbs. Among the types of activity that are monitored with biofeedback instruments are muscle or electromyographic (EMG) activity, changes in blood flow as measured through skin temperature, changes in EEG or brain wave activity, and changes in skin response (sweating), which tracks emotions or moods. Feedback is also used to monitor heart rate, respiration, gastrointestinal activity, and sphincters that control movement of substances from one part of the gastrointestinal tract to another.

Biofeedback, which is used as an adjunct with other therapies, such as medication and physiotherapy, is developing into a versatile and useful therapy. More than ten thousand papers have been published demonstrating the effectiveness of biofeedback for the management of more than 150 medical and psychological disorders.

Why does it work?

The most common explanation is that you become increasingly expert at discriminating internal body cues and adjusting your senses and muscles to them.

Neal Miller, Ph.D., professor emeritus and former head of a laboratory of physiological psychology at Rockefeller University in New York, is the father of biofeedback. He maintains that through biofeedback it is now obvious that the mind cannot direct the activities of the body unless it has information about what is going on in the environment of the body, its tissues, and its cells. And we should have known that if the brain cannot operate without information from the body, and the body cannot operate without information from the brain, then both are not merely connected, they exist and function as a unit.

Dr. Miller says that most of us can control what we do with arms and legs, with eye and face and other muscles, using the kind of body control called voluntary. But until recently, medical science believed and taught that nearly all our other body functions, such as blood flow, body temperature, brain waves, or even residual muscle tension itself, were under automatic regulation and beyond our control.[17]

Many other successful clinical applications of biofeedback, besides Dr. Miller's report, were presented at the 1985 Biofeedback Society of America meeting in New Orleans, Louisiana. Among them:

Patients with Raynaud's disease—a disorder of the blood vessels in which exposure to the cold causes the small arteries supplying the fingers and toes to contract suddenly, cutting off blood flow to the digits, which then become pale and painful—learned to raise the temperature in their hands through biofeedback at Wayne State University. These patients were thus able to reduce their constriction attacks by 93 percent over a three-year period.[18]

Diabetics with leg and foot ulcers that would not heal were taught to raise the temperature of the affected limb and thus increase the blood supply. Two out of three patients at the Veterans Administration Hospital in Salt Lake City were able to induce healing of diabetic foot ulcers with the aid of biofeedback.[19]

Six insulin-taking diabetics were taught to relax more effectively with biofeedback techniques at Georgetown Univeristy in Washington, D.C. As a result, they had decreased blood-glucose levels, required less insulin, and had fewer incidences of great blood-sugar fluctuations.[20]

Patients with strabismus (crossed eyes or lazy eyes) were taught to control eye movement by biofeedback tones at the University of the Pacific, Forest Grove, Oregon. They typically had a failure of the neural control circuits that point and coordinate the eyes. When an eye deviates inward or outward, the brain is forced to deal with separate images from the two eyes. This can produce double vision, and the brain often corrects this problem by suppressing the output from one of the eyes, thus wasting its output. The patients learned to keep their eyes straight for two minutes in the dark or while viewing a blank white field.[21]

Three patients with elevated inner-eye pressure—a condition that can cause blindness—were taught relaxation techniques through biofeedback at the University of Alabama in Birmingham. They achieved reduced intraocular pressure, probably because they reduced muscle tension around the eye. The researchers are continuing their investigation of the result.[22]

A fifty-seven-year-old patient, incapacitated with cerebral palsy, was taught through biofeedback to control involuntary movements—jerking, twitching, tremor, and muscle spasms—through biofeedback. After a few months, he was able to dress himself, tie his own shoe laces, and walk eight to ten blocks. With fewer involuntary movements and less spasticity, he was able to fish from a boat and to climb stairs unaided, all of which he could not do before.[23]

Twelve girls with curvature of the spine, which would normally have required a body brace, were taught through the use of a halter that caused a bell to sound when they did not stand straight to correct the curvature. Ten out of the twelve were able to avoid the brace.[24]

Biofeedback is also being used to train a person's brain to control its own brain waves. Two papers were presented at the Biofeedback Society's meeting in Louisiana that concerned training children with learning disabilities to overcome deficits with brain-wave biofeedback.

Union, New Jersey, psychologist, Michael Tansey, Ph.D., reported that he is training learning-disabled children to exercise the brain circuitry of their sensorimotor cortex (learning centers). Once aware of this brain-wave rhythm, they attempt to increase it. "Thus," Dr. Tansey said, "the brain may be viewed as a biological computer, the mind as a medium through which to access a cerebral exercise program with the electroencephalograph as a monitor, and the individual as a now-informed programmer."

Dr. Tansey claims that brain-wave training results in improved hand-eye coordination, cessation of erratic eye movements, improved fine motor control in general and increased attentional flexibility, positive academic advancement through greater information processing ability and memory capabilities, and increased IQ scores.[25]

Joel Lubar, Ph.D., of the University of Tennessee, and Judith Lubar, M.A., of the Southeastern Biofeedback Institute, reported at the same meeting that they recorded and analyzed the difference between the EEGs from the brains of 150 normal and learning-disabled children. Then through EEG biofeedback, they helped the learning-disabled youngsters to develop a more normal pattern. The youngsters attempted to increase the fast brain-wave activity associated with concentration and attention and at the same time to inhibit the slow brain-wave activity and undesirable muscle activity, which might interfere with learning and concentration.[26]

Communicating directly with brain waves may also be possible, according to a report at the same meeting given by S. Thomas Elder, Ph.D., of the University of New Orleans, and his colleagues. They reported that their ultimate goal is to develop a method to allow patients suffering from the degenerative disease amyotrophic lateral sclerosis (Lou Gehrig's disease), who are unable to move or speak but who can think, to communicate their needs. Through biofeedback, the researchers succeeded in teaching four volunteers to produce certain brain waves that caused a device to sound one tone for "yes" and another for "no" in response to questions.[27]

It is not surprising, therefore, that biofeedback has been successful with insomniacs and with migraine-headache sufferers. The former are taught to relax and allow sleep to arrive; the latter, how to raise the temperature in their hands to dilate blood vessels in spasm. In migraine, it is the blood vessels in the brain that dilate and cause pain. The body is designed to sacrifice blood flow to any other area in order to preserve blood flow to the brain. Therefore, the blood vessels in the hands constrict to shunt blood to the dilated blood vessels in the head during a migraine attack. As the hands are warmed, the blood vessels in them dilate and help, by a sort of reflex action, reduce the flow of blood to the brain. This also works for patients with Raynaud's syndrome.

Ease-a-Pain with Temperature Feedback

If you have a headache or pain elsewhere in your body, mark the intensity from 1 to 10 on the scale on the next page. Hold an ordinary fever, meat, or household thermometer in your hand and place your elbow in a bowl or sinkfull of cold water. Wait two minutes and note the temperature on the thermometer. Then put your elbow in a bowl of warm water, about 100° to 103° F, and concentrate on the thermometer. Will your hand to get warmer and warmer. See if you can raise the mercury by at least one degree. Wait for five minutes and then write down the current intensity of your pain on the scale. Did it ease? With practice, you may greatly relieve your discomfort by this biofeedback, hand-warming method.

The fact that you can "think" your hand warm is quite remarkable. No one is absolutely certain exactly how the brain and body work together to achieve this. However, it is believed that reward may be a large factor. You know that when you are trying to achieve something and you are cheered on or receive information that you are getting closer to your goal, you press onward. The information is a reward and helps you to keep trying until you succeed.

Do Your Own Biofeedback

Buying yourself a present when you've accomplished something that was difficult is a form of biofeedback. Looking at yourself naked in the mirror when your are on a diet is another form of biofeedback.

If you have access to a blood pressure apparatus, the result of your trying consciously to lower your blood pressure may show you some remarkable results. It takes relaxation, repetition, and the will to do it, along with the feedback from the numbers on the gauge.

EASE-A-PAIN TEMPERATURE SCALE									
Day I		Day II		Day III		Day IV		Day V	
Before	After	Before	After	Before	After	Before	After	Before	After
10									
9									
8									
7									
6									
5									
4									
3									
2									
1									

Hypnosis

Hypnosis is an older method of mind over matter and stress-reduction. The word *hypnosis* is derived from the name of the Greek god of sleep, Hypnos. While similar to sleep, hypnosis is actually a state of consciousness in which you are highly open to suggestion. In heterohypnosis, another person suggests the images, and in self-hypnosis, you do.

In order to experience hypnosis, there must be a sense of immediate involvement in one's mental imagery and detachment from the surrounding external environment. A variety of physiological and emotional states can be aroused or calmed. Hypnotic suggestions can be made in relation to the sensations of taste, touch, smell, and sight. Suggestions (known as posthypnotic) can also be made concerning expectations about forthcoming events. The physiologic explanation of how and why hypnosis works to relieve stress and pain is yet to be made.[28] However, since the right side of the brain is concerned with diffuse, holistic, and intuitive thought and action, while the left brain is devoted more to analytic thinking, hypnosis is probably a right-brain phenomenon.

Indeed, when University of Washington researchers studied the brain waves of patients having wisdom teeth removed with hypnosis as the only anesthesia, the investigators found the dental patients' EEGs showed more activity on the right side of the brain.[29]

Drs. Ernest and Josephine Hilgard of Stanford University, two of the world's leading experts in the field, believe that human consciousness "flows" in more than one channel. That is, our awareness can take place at more than one level at the same time. Disassociation of the levels of our awareness occurs quite naturally. For instance, when we learn complex skills such as driving a car, we find initially that we have to pay full attention to each part of the task. As we become more expert, we can think of other things while driving and even talk to our companions. There is a wide variation in the ease with which people experience hypnosis but nearly everyone can. Those most difficult to hypnotize are the highly intellectual who constantly analyze and find it difficult to accept suggestions and the unintelligent who have little control over their conscious mind. The best subjects are those with average intelligence and a good imagination.[30]

Hypnotize Yourself

Exercise 1. Sit in a chair and look at a spot on the wall. Tell yourself that your eyelids are heavy, very heavy—so heavy you can't keep them open. Close your eyes slowly. Take five deep, slow breaths. Let your shoulders relax, then your abdomen relax, then your knees relax so they're apart. Tell yourself that your right arm is heavy, very heavy—so heavy that you can't hold it up. Keep concentrating on your right arm until you feel it is heavy. Then open your eyes and you will be able to just concentrate on your right arm and by association feel relaxed immediately. And you will be able to perform this autosuggestion relaxation anywhere, and at any time.

Exercise 2. Sit comfortably in a chair and do progressive relaxation. Tense the muscles of your toes for the count of four, and relax for the count of four. Tense your calf muscles for the count of four and relax for the count of four. Continue tensing and relaxing your muscles all the way up to your forehead.

When you have finished, look straight ahead at the wall and try to keep your eyes open without blinking for the count of fifty. (Don't you feel compelled to blink?)

Exercise 3. Think about your nose itching. Tell yourself over and over that it itches and that you must scratch it. Keep thinking about it for two minutes—your nose tickles and you have to scratch it.

If you blinked or scratched your nose, you are in a state of suggestibility. Now, repeat the relaxation exercise and then tell yourself in one phrase something you wish to accomplish, such as: "I am not going to let my boss upset me" or "I am going to win that tennis game tomorrow."

Repeat the phrase fifteen times while keeping your body relaxed. Eventually, you will be able to hypnotize yourself effectively without the relaxation exercises.

Meditate

If you think meditation is only a religious or a "hippie" practice, think again. It is a "time out" to lower your stress level and prepare you for what you have to do. Just sit in a comfortable chair with your eyes closed and concentrate on your breathing for a few minutes. Then begin silently to repeat a mantra, a meaningless word such as "ommmmm." Imagine your whole body resonating with the quiet sound of this word. As the relaxation response, you should gently banish intruding thoughts by concentrating on your personal mantra.

Massage Yourself

As you learned in this book, touch is reflected in your brain. Massaging yourself is not only relaxing, it is good for your brain. You send signals from you hands and skin to your brain and, in turn, your brain tells your muscles to relax. Massage improves circulation and sensation and generally enhances your well-being, especially if you use an oil with a scent that you find pleasant.

Smile and Benefit Your Brain

Hypnosis, of course, is a mental exercise that can affect the physiology of both brain and body. But can exercising the facial muscles to portray classic emotions also affect the physiology of the brain?

The theory that facial expressions affect brain function was first suggested more than eighty years ago by Israel Waynbaum, M.D., in a book published in Paris, *Physionomie humaine: Son mechanisme et son role social.* Dr. Waynbaum maintained that all emotional reactions produce circulatory changes and affect blood flow to the brain. Smiling and laughing, the major expressions of happiness, increase blood flow and oxygen to the brain, while expressions of depression curb blood flow. The tears shed during hard laughter are nature's way of releasing pressure in the brain built up by the laughing.

If you find this hard to believe, look in the mirror. Put your fingers in your mouth and pull your lips into an exaggerated smile. Hold the expression for the count of one hundred. Look at the artery in your forehead. It should be pulsing noticeably because the muscles you are pulling act to impede the blood flow into the face and thus increase the pressure of blood in your brain.

Why do you furrow your brow when concentrating? By tightening the muscles in your forehead, you delay the flow of blood from the brain and allow the organ more nourishment for its harder work.

R. B. Zjonc, professor of psychology at the University of Michigan, points out that if brain temperature can influence moods by facilitating the release of particular neurotransmitters, and if facial musculature can modify brain temperature, then control of the appropriate facial muscles can induce more favorable moods. Yoga and various forms of meditation are based in part on such assumptions. Whether deliberate expressions have the same effectiveness as spontaneous ones is still to be proven.[31]

So there are many methods under investigation that can provide a greater understanding and control over stress. Biofeedback, hypnosis, and other relaxation techniques are widely used, effective aids. However, ultimately, the control over your own stress reactions is up to you.

It may require changes in your lifestyle. Some of the alterations may be quite simple and others very difficult.

The following are techniques that have evolved over the years and have proved successful in alleviating stress. They are based on two approaches:

1. Controlling the sources of stress more effectively
2. Creating a drain to relieve the tension.

Identify Your Stressors

Write Down Your Major Source(s) of Stress at Home _____

_____

_____

Write Down Your Major Source(s) of Stress at Work _____

_____

_____

Write Down Your Major Source(s) of Stress in Your Social Life ___

_____

_____

Write Down How You Deal with the Stresses That Occasionally Come Up and at Least Three Ideas of How You Could Better Cope with the Stressors (you can discuss the ideas with friends or relatives) _____

_____

_____

The As and Bs of Stress. You have identified your stressors above. Now make an A list and a B list. Under the As, list those stressors over which you have some measure of control. Under the B list identify those things over which you have no control. Once you have written the two lists, tear up the B list and concentrate on the A list. Now, using numbers—one being the top priority—identify those stressors that need to be dealt with first. Then under the top-priority things, come up with at least three possible solutions. They can be nonsensical or realistic, but thinking about them will help you eventually deal with the problem.

Write a Letter. You will not send it, but put down exactly how you feel about the stressor. If the issue is doing the dishes or if it is the way your mate or mother behaves at a particular time, vent all your feelings. Put down all the horrible things you wanted to say but never did.

Accept Yourself. Tell yourself that everyone has mean thoughts and that if you bury them, they don't go away. They fester. Pamper yourself. If you get enough rest and relaxation, you'll be better able to cope. It is better to have a high opinion of yourself and be accused of being egotistical than a low opinion of yourself and find that others accept your own evaluation. That's the road to depression and stress. If you love yourself, you'll be able to be more loving to others.[32]

Don't Be a Martyr. Learn to delegate responsibility. Training and motivating others to do tasks customarily performed by you can reduce your time burdens in the future. That's true at home and at work.

Think About Communication. If you have never resolved your conflicts from your childhood, perhaps it is time to reveal what you really feel. You don't have to put people on the defensive by saying, "You make me so mad when . . ." or "I don't like it when you . . ." Instead, be open and say, "I wish you'd do it differently because . . ." or "Consider my feelings when thin . . ." and let the person know in a nice way how his or her actions affect you.

Make a Decision. It is better to make the wrong decision than to avoid making a decision at all. You have to decide now whether it will be A or B. Anybody can think of good reasons on both sides. But if you wait for 100 percent assurance, you'll wait forever. So make up your mind. Make the decision and carry it out. An error can be corrected, but indecision that causes stress can damage your brain and body.

Don't Overdo Details. Details can be completed, but sometimes a concern about small things leads to smallness in thinking. Some people become tense because they drown in their own details and then get pulled every which way worrying about them.

Prioritize. Set realistic goals and priorities, and identify those things you must do first. Organize your time in accordance with those priorities.

Don't Insist on Winning. Everybody loses sometime and you are no different from anyone else. Sometimes we benefit more by losing and trying again than by winning.

Don't Wait for the Sword to Fall. If you are anxious about something and you can't talk yourself out of the anxiety, try to advance the event that is making you tense so that the anticipated occasion comes and goes in your mind. Note that you survived the event and think about that the next time you are worried about a future occurrence.

Identify Your Goals

	TOMORROW	ONE YEAR	TEN YEARS
WORK			
PERSONAL			

Exercise—The Instant Stress Reliever

Exercise is one of the best stress relievers. If you can, just walk away from a stressful situation. A fifteen-minute walk will do wonders for taking you away from the source of stress and getting your breathing deeper and more regular and the blood flowing.

If you are in an office—your own or someone else's—and you feel stressed, shrug your shoulders. Tension is usually first felt in the your shoulders and neck.

Gently shrug your shoulders up and back three times and then up and forward three times.

Bend your chin slowly and gently to your chest. Raise it up to the starting position and then slowly and gently bend your head back. Do this three times.

Turn your head slowly to one shoulder. Back to the front, and then look over the other shoulder. Do this three times.

And finally:

Get Sufficient Sleep. Find your own personal sleep needs— whether it is four or ten hours a night. No one's brain works right when the body is fatigued.

Learn to Say No. When you feel stressed and overloaded with obligations, just say no. You owe it to yourself to stop stress damage, and your brain will work better when you can say yes.

Relax As Soon As You Are Fatigued. If you wait until you are completely exhausted, you will be tense and it will be more difficult for you to recuperate.

Remember That Sex May Be Good for Your Brain. Studies have shown that sexual stimulation releases endorphins in the brain and not only eases tension but relieves the pain of arthritis and other ailments. Animal studies have shown that stimulation of the genitals increases brain metabolism.[33] So, if you need a good excuse to have sex, there it is. Sex will help you think better.

Know When You Need to Use Relaxation Exercises. When you are anxious, feel overburdened, and feel tension mounting, STOP, take three deep breaths, and use one or more of the techniques you have learned in this chapter. In fact, to prevent stress from overcoming you, take ten minutes every day to employ one of the relaxation exercises.

Stop Making Excuses. As we have described repeatedly, your brain has amazing powers that remain vital if you continue to exercise them well into old age. Don't concentrate on the "if onlys" and the "I would have, buts." You can't change your parents, the place of your birth, your brothers and sisters, or your talents—but you can make the most of what you've got. Take action!

13

Do You Need Professional Help?

How do you know when your brain or the brain of some significant other person in your life is not just "flabby" and "unexercised" but in need of a professional diagnosis?

As pointed out in this book, there are many things that can interfere with your brain that can be corrected, from just plain disuse to side effects of drugs and stress. According to the U.S. Department of Health and Human Services, more than seventy conditions affecting at least three to four million Americans can cause a loss of intellectual abilities. It has been determined that as much as 20 percent of the people diagnosed with Alzheimer's do not have it. Instead of being considered hopeless, many of these people may have conditions that are reversible, such as Parkinson's disease or depression that will respond well to medication. Even nutritional deficiencies have been found to cause severe memory problems.

No book can replace a thorough diagnosis by a physician, but here are some questions that may lead you in the right direction.

Answer True or False

I CAN REMEMBER SOMETHING THAT HAPPENED YEARS AGO BUT NOT WHERE I PUT MY KEYS. _____

Answer: Most people over forty years old will answer True. The reason is probably because there is so much going on in your life at the time you weren't paying attention when you put your keys away.

I CAN'T REMEMBER THE NAME OF SOMEONE I KNEW VERY WELL IN THE PAST. _____

Answer: Again, most of us will answer True. *It is a question of re-trieval—finding the name where it is filed in your memory bank. The name usually pops up if you don't try too hard.*

I OPEN THE REFRIGERATOR AND CAN'T REMEMBER WHAT I WANTED. _____

Answer: Again, most people—even those in their twenties—will answer True. *It is usually a result of interference from other thoughts or dis-tractions.*

I AM HAVING TROUBLE BECAUSE I FORGET CALLS I WAS SUPPOSED TO MAKE OR REPORTS THAT WERE DUE. _____

Answer: If you answer True *to this one and it is interfering with your work or your family life, you should seek a physical examination and, if necessary, a memory evaluation.*

I GET MORE IRRITATED OR ANNOYED THAN I USED TO. _____

Answer: If you answered True, *you may be in an emotional state that interferes with your intellectual functioning and you should seek pro-fessional help.*

I BEGAN HAVING TROUBLE AFTER A CHANGE IN A RELA-TIONSHIP OR THE START OF A NEW MEDICATION. _____

Answer: If you answered True, *you may have an emotional problem or you may have been given a medication that has a side effect that inter-feres with memory function. This is very common and can easily be remedied, so check with your physician.*

I'M DRIVING MY CAR OR WALKING DOWN A STREET AND I SUDDENLY GET CONFUSED ABOUT WHERE I AM OR HOW I GOT THERE. _____

Answer: This may be a sign of a serious problem if you answered True, *and warrants a complete checkup by professionals.*

WHEN SOMEONE IS JUST INTRODUCED TO ME, I CAN'T RE-MEMBER THEIR NAME TWO MINUTES LATER. _____

Answer: Most of us do not really listen when introduced to someone, so a True *answer is almost universal because we do not concentrate when we are told the name.*

I HAVE DIFFICULTY MAKING DECISIONS RECENTLY.

_____

Answer: A True *answer to this again means that you may be in an emotional or physical state that interferes with intellectual function, and warrants a thorough physical and emotional checkup.*

I FORGET TO TURN OFF THE STOVE OR TO LOCK THE DOOR. _____

Answer: If you answer True *to this one, you may endanger your life or the lives of your loved ones and you should have a memory evaluation. It could just be carelessness, the side effect of medication, or emotional upset.*

THESE SYMPTOMS, WITHOUT A DOUBT, REQUIRE PROMPT DIAGNOSIS!

- Getting lost in familiar surroundings and not recognizing something that before was common in the environment, such as keys or kitchen appliances.
- Loss of comprehension.
- Having problems with routine tasks.
- Significant changes in personality and judgment.
- Agitation.
- Feeling distrustful of everyone.
- Not being able to recognize members of your family or friends.
- Difficulty with speaking or loss of speech.
- Major changes in appetite and weight loss.
- Inability to control bladder or bowel movements.
- Frequent repetition of stories without being aware of it.

What to Expect from a Neurological Examination

The earlier a diagnosis is made, the better the chance for intervening and preventing further deterioration—even in the cases of Alzheimer's disease. The first step in diagnosis is a thorough medical history, including past illnesses, current eating habits, lifestyle, and mood. Obtaining a history may be difficult in a patient with a memory problem, however. If the patient is confused and unable to answer simple questions regarding such things as the day, time, and current U.S. president, then the physician must rely on family, caregivers, and medical records from a physician or hospital for the medical history.

You may undergo screening tests such as the Mini-Mental State (MMS), which evaluates a broad range of cognitive functions such as orientation, recall, attention, calculation, language, manipulation, and constructional ability. There are a number of other such tests, including computerized testing.

The next step is to differentiate between psychological and organic disorders. Again, tests may be used to determine depression and concentration. Often in the case of elderly persons, results of such tests may be skewed because the questions are more appropriate for younger persons; however, new tests are being developed.

If the physician finds a person has significant memory loss, then further tests are required. Among them are laboratory and psychological tests. If these tests are abnormal, then even further tests are recommended. These may include:

- **EEG** (Electroencephalograph). Records the electrical activity from the brain. Advanced version of it is known as the BEAM (brain electrical activity mapping) or the Brain Mapper, which is a diagram display of the brain activity.

- **CAT Scan** (Computerized axial tomography). A scanner that uses X-rays to visualize the brain in cross section. Computer screens then display "slices" of the brain viewed from any desired angle. It shows the anatomy of the brain and is used to diagnose strokes, bleeding, swelling, and lesions.

- **MRI** (Magnetic resonance imaging). Does not involve X-ray or other radiation. It provides a high-quality, detailed, three-dimensional image of the brain.

- **MRS** (Magnetic resonance spectroscopy). This uses the same equipment as the MRI with an added technique that enables a physician to examine chemistry rather than anatomy.
- **MRA** (Magnetic resonance angiography). Produces an image of the arteries and veins of the brain.
- **MSI** (Magnetic source imaging). This machine reveals the weak magnetic fields emitted by nerve cells firing electrical signals. By tracking the magnetic fields, scientists can determine the origin of epileptic seizures and responses to sound, touch, and vision.
- **SPECT Scan** (Single photon emitting tomography). Reveals normal and abnormal blood flow in the brain and aids in the diagnosis of stroke and Alzheimer's.
- **PET Scan** (Photo emitting tomography). This shows the function of the brain and sites for thinking, vision, and hearing via the brain's use of blood sugar.

Since there are reversible conditions that masquerade as Alzheimer's and other brain degenerative diseases, proper diagnosis is vital. A complete and thorough examination should identify the cause of memory loss. Then either the loss can be reversed by appropriate therapy or further progression of memory loss may be prevented or delayed. Among the therapies available:

- **Computerized biofeedback training.** Uses include therapy for migraine headaches, anxiety/tension, high blood pressure, Raynaud's vasospasm, paralysis, and cognitive stimulation.
- **Cognitive rehabilitation.** Brain exercises to improve memory that are used as therapy for post-concussion syndrome, movement control, and concept deficiencies. May include speech therapy, computerized programs, and psychotherapy.
- **Medications.** These are given according to diagnosis and symptoms. The antidepressants, anti-Parkinson medications, antianxiety drugs, supplementary nutrition, multivitamins, vitamins E and B-12 (intramuscular), and medications for early Alzheimer's, such as Tacrine and Hydergine. (Other, more effective medications for Alzheimer's are expected on the market as of this writing.)

14

Prepare for Your Future

With your eyes shut, picture a bottle.
Turn the bottle upside down.
Make it smaller.
Make it larger.
Change the shape of it.
Change the color of it.
Bring it as close to you as you can.
Open your eyes! You have now demonstrated the marvelous things only your brain can do.

You have the ability to perform better, to use more of your potential, and to be a happier, more effective person.

As we have pointed out throughout this book, great progress has already been made in understanding the brain and its effect on body functions and the body's effect on the brain. It has been proven that the continued development of your brain is not significantly limited by your age. The potential is there. You can learn to handle environmental stress so that it does not damage your brain and body. You can gain greater control over the stimulation your brain receives and the signals it puts out. There is one thing that both the computer and the brain require—an input to produce an output. Too often, in our culture, we stop inputting a lot of new data into our brains after a certain age.

• Ella Tuttle Mattheson, a 102-year-old columnist for the *Clinton*, a newspaper in Clinton, Michigan, maintains: "My memory is as sharp today as it ever was. It's just that I have to tax it a little more. But then, I've got a lot more to remember than anyone else."[1]

• Philip L. Carret, who helped to give birth to the mutual fund industry, was, as of this writing, still working forty hours a week as a stockbroker, doing his own cooking, and writing his fourth book, "The Patient Investor." He is scheduled to celebrate his one hundredth birthday in November.[2]

• James Michener, at ninety years and on kidney dialysis, completed a book in 1996 and in a television interview said he had four more books that he was planning to write. His body may have been weakening, but his mind and his creativity were absolutely intact.

• Dorothy Fuldheim, a legendary Midwest broadcaster in her ninth decade, put it succinctly: "It gets my goat when people say it's remarkable how bright I am at my age. I was bright forty years ago. And the more I use my brain, the sharper it gets."[3]

We couldn't agree more. Your brain has a tremendous capacity.

A computer is a wondrous—if sometimes frustrating machine. It can remember millions of bits of information and if you press the right keys, it will recall a specific bit of data. But the computer cannot really think. It cannot recognize the face of someone at a twenty-fifth class reunion who put on weight, lost his hair, and only vaguely resembles his former self. Even though your brain retains the old image, it can still deal with the changes and recognize your old classmates.

Raymond Truex and Malcolm Carpenter pointed out in their text *Human Anatomy:*

> "Electronic brains" are impressive in appearance and function; yet they do not approach in versatility or scope the fantastic potentialities of the human brain. The human brain is unique in that it can provide its own programming; in fact, it is programmed throughout life by our daily experience. It seems likely that "electronic brains" will in the future perform many more of the functions now performed by human brains, but this change must be regarded as a redistribution of labor, not a replacement. The "electronic brain" is after all only one of the many expressions of the ingenuity of the human brain.[4]

The future of human brain research is nearly beyond imagination. As the neurosciences progress, it will be possible to further project and enhance brain function. Successful transplantation of brain tissue will be accomplished and disabilities overcome. There will soon be drugs to strengthen failing memories and to increase concentration. The riddles of the chemical aberrations that cause schizophrenia and autism will be solved.

Today's advanced technology permits probing inside the living brain to interpret function. Neuroscientists can see metabolism and flow as related to function. Researchers at the Weizmann Institute in Rehovot, Israel, report that by monitoring the internal patterns of activity of a person's brain, they are able for the first time to predict the exact brain-wave patterns evoked by a visual image. Moreover, they are able to tell what simple picture the eyes had just seen. Such neuroscientists are just beginning to literally "read" our minds.

They may be able to tell what we are seeing and thinking, but they cannot determine creativity nor evaluate finite potential. They cannot measure motivation.[5]

What you do with your brain—how you challenge it and exercise it to keep it in top form and achieving its full potential—well, that's all in your head!

Notes

1. You Can Gain Brain Power

1. Henry H. Donaldson, *The Growth of the Brain: A Study of the Nervous System in Relation to Education* (New York: Scribner's, 1895).
2. Steven Petersen, Ph.D., and Randy Buckner, Washington University, St. Louis, Mo., "Men from Mars, Women from Venus Use Same Parts of the Brain to Generate Words," paper presented at the Society for Neuroscience's annual meeting, November 1994, Miami, Fla.
3. Gina Kolata, "Man's World, Woman's World? Brain Studies Point to Differences," *New York Times*, Feb. 28, 1995, p. C1.
4. Ranjan Duara, M.D., interview with authors, National Institutes of Health, Bethesda, Md., April 13, 1984.
5. Senility Reconsidered: Treatment Possibilities for Mental Impairment in the Elderly," Task Force sponsored by the National Institute on Aging, Bethesda, Md., *Journal of the American Medical Association*, July 18, 1980, 259–60; R. Dura, M.D., et al., "Cerebral Glucose Utilization as Measured with Positron Emission Tomography in 21 Resting Healthy Men Between the Ages of 21 and 83 Years," *Brain*, 106 (1983): 761–75; K. Warner Schaie, ed., *Longitudinal Studies of Adult Psychological Development* (New York: Guilford Press, 1983); Marian Cleeves Diamond, Ph.D., and James R. Connor, Department of Physiology, University of California at Berkeley, paper presented at the Tenth Annual Meeting of the Society for Neuroscience, Cincinnati, Ohio, Nov. 9–10, 1980; Ruth Winter, "Biomarkers: Beating Body Burnout," *American Health*, May 1984: 70–80; Mark R. Rosenzweig, Ph.D., and Edward Bennett, Ph.D., University of California, Lawrence Berkeley Laboratory, June 24, 1980, "The Physiological Imprint of Learning," U.S. Department of Health Research Grant

Report, National Institutes of Health, May 1986; John Sladek, Jr., Ph.D., and Carol Phelps, Ph.D., paper presented at the International Catecholamine Symposium, Göteborg, Sweden, June 12, 1983.

6. National Institute of Medicine Report, Washington, D.C., March 31, 1981.

7. Winter, op. cit.

8. Bernice Grafstein, Cornell University Medical College, speech presented to the Society for Neuroscience Writers Seminar, New York, Nov. 9, 1976; Carmelita Frondoza, Reinhard Grzanna, and Richard Humphrey, "Effects of 6-Hydroxydopamine and Reserpine on the Growth of LPC-1 Plasmacytoma," paper presented at the Annual Meeting of the Society for Neuroscience, Boston, Mass., Nov. 7, 1983; T. G. Saith, Jr., M.D., Laboratory of Neurophysiology, paper presented at the Society for Neuroscience meeting, Atlanta, Ga., Nov. 6, 1979.

9. Sladek and Phelps, op. cit.

10. Diamond, op. cit.

11. Ibid.—Diamond, op cit.

12. Shaie, op. cit.; Rosenzweig and Bennett, op. cit.

13. Michael R. Sperling, "Temporal Lobectomy for Refractory Epilepsy," *Journal of the American Medical Association*, August 14, 1996, 276 (6): 470–75.

14. Elizabeth A. McCusker, M.B., B.S., et al., "Recovery from Locked-In Syndrome," *Archives of Neurology*, 39 (3)(March 1983): 145–47.

15. Joan O'Connor, "Research Using Head-Injured Vietnam Veterans Shows Effects of Brain Lesions on Mental Performance," *Psychiatric News*, May 17, 1985.

16. Ruth Levine, "Reorganizing the Brain," *Touchstone*, 18(3), University of Wisconsin-Madison Research Program (December 1984).

17. O'Connor, op. cit.

18. Claudia Kawas, M.D., associate professor of neurology at Johns Hopkins Medical Institutions, in a speech at the American Association for the Advancement of Science, February 12, 1996, Baltimore, Md.

19. World Health Organization's *Treatise on Neuroplasticity and Repair in the Central Nervous System* (Geneva, Switzerland, 1983).

2. Sense and Sensitivity

1. Philip Solomon, "Sensory Deprivation: Its Meaning and Significance," *State of Mind*, Ciba Publication, November 1958.

2. Ibid.

3. Ibid.

4. Ashley Montagu, *Touching: The Human Significance of the Skin* (New York: Perennial, 1972).

5. John Kubie, et al., Downstate Medical Center, Brooklyn, NY, "Manipulations of the Geometry of Environmental Enclosures Control the Spatial Firing Patterns of Hippocampal Neurons," paper presented at the Society for Neuroscience meeting, Boston, Mass., Nov. 9, 1983.

6. Stephen K. Itaya, Ph.D., "Retinal Inputs to Limbic Auditory and Motor Areas in the Rat," paper presented at the Society for Neuroscience meeting, Cincinnati, Ohio, Nov. 9, 1980.

7. Yogi Berra, and Tom Horton, *Yogi: It Ain't Over . . .* (McGraw-Hill Publishing Company, New York: McGraw-Hill, 1989).

8. Mark Rosensweig, Ph.D., David Krech, Ph.D., and Marian Diamond, Ph.D., "The Physiological Imprint of Learning Investigators," paper prepared by Gay Luce after interviews in December 1965 and May 1966, National Institutes of Health publication.

9. David Hubel, and Torsten Wiesel, "Respective Fields, Binocular Interation, and Functional Architecture in a Cat's Visual Cortex," *Journal of Physiology* (London) 160 (1962): 106–54; and "Shape and Arrangement of Columns in a Cat's Striate Cortex," *Journal of Physiology* (London) 165 (1962–63): 559–68.

10. Donald Kline, Ph.D., associate professor of psychology, University of Notre Dame, Notre Dame, Ind., report of National Institutes of Health's Research Career Development, March 16, 1984.

11. Jane Brody, "Surprising Health Impact Discovered for Light," *New York Times*, Nov. 13, 1984, p. C1.

12. "How Today's Noise Hurts Body and Mind," *Medical World News*, June 13, 1969, 42–43.

13. M. D. Safranek, "Effect of Auditory Rhythm on Muscle Reactivity," *Physical Therapy*, February 1982, 161–88.

14. *Medical World News*, op. cit.

15. Ruth Winter, "Music: The New Active Sport," *Self*, May 1984, 175.

16. Ruth Winter, *The Smell Book* (New York: J. P. Lippincott, 1978).

17. R. C. Trux, et al., *Human Neuroanatomy* (Baltimore, MD.: Williams and Wilkins, 1964).

18. Susan Schiffman, Ph.D., "Taste and Smell in Disease (Part One)," *New England Journal of Medicine*, 308 (21) (May 26, 1983): 1275–79 and "Taste and Smell in Disease (Part Two)," *New England Journal of Medicine*, 308 (22) (June 2, 1983): 1337–43.

19. Rita Schul, "Unforgettable Flavors: Flavor Memory Site Identi-

fied in Weizmann Institute Study," paper presented at Society for Neurosciences Meeting, San Diego, Ca, Nov. 15, 1995.

20. James Weifeenbach, Ph.D., ed., "Taste and Development: The Genesis of Sweet Preference," National Institute of Dental Research, U.S. Department of Health, Bethesda, Md., 1977, No. (ADM) 75–236.

21. Michael Curley, Ph.D., and Robert Hawkins, Ph.D., "Cognitive Performance During a Heat Acclimatization Regimen," *Aviation Space Environmental Medicine* (August 1983): 709–13.

3. Enhancing Coordination and Motor Skills

1. Jeff Harrison, "Motor Control," *Report on Research: Neuroscience,* University of Arizona, Tucson, Summer–Fall 1989, vol. 6, number 1, p. 9–11.

2. E. V. Evarts, "Brain Mechanisms in Voluntary Movements," *Scientific American,* September 1979, 164–79; Carol Phelps, and John Sladek, Department of Anatomy, University of Rochester, "Regeneration of Central Catecholamine Fibers in Aged Rates," paper presented at the Society of Neuroscience meeting, Boston, Mass., Nov. 10, 1983; Walter Kroll, University of Massachusetts, interview with author, October 1984, and various papers; K. V. Anderson, et al., "Neuromuscular Control Mechanism in Oromotor Behavior," paper presented at the Society for Neuroscience meeting, Anaheim, Calif., Oct. 11, 1984.

3. R. J. Nelson, et al., "Variations in the Proportional Representation of the Hand in Somatosensory Cortex of Primates," paper presented at the Society for Neuroscience meeting, Boston, Mass., Nov. 13, 1980.

4. W. M. Jenkins, M. M. Merzenich, and M. T. Ochs, Coleman Memorial Labs, Department of Otolaryngology and Physiology, University of California at San Francisco, paper presented at the Society for Neuroscience Meeting, Anaheim, Calif., Oct. 13, 1984.

5. Kroll, op. cit.

6. Angela Sirigu, Jean-Rene Duhamel, et al., "The Mental Representation of Hand Movements After Parietal Cortex Damage," *Science,* vol. 273, September 13, 1996, p. 1564–67.

7. Yogi Berra, and Tom Horton, *Yogi: It Ain't Over . . .* (New York: McGraw-Hill Publishing Co., 1989).

8. "Brain Facts: A Primer on the Brain and Nervous System," Society for Neuroscience, Washington, D.C., 1990, p. 18.

9. "Special Report on Aging," February 1980, and Seminar for Science Writers, Bethesda, Md., January 1981.

10. Mark Williams, M.D., University of Rochester, interview with author, April 1984.

11. Special Report on Aging, U.S. Department of Health, NIH Publication No. 80-2135, August 1980.

4. Brain Aerobics

1. F. Chaouloff, "Physical Exercise and Brain Monoamines: A Review," *Acta Physology Scandinavia* 1989, 137, 1–3.

2. Charles Ransford, "A Role for Amines in the Antidepressant Effect of Exercise: A Review," *Medicine and Science in Sports and Exercise,* 12 (1) (1982): 1–10.

3. B. S. Brown, et al., "Chronic Response of Rat Brain Norepinephrine and Serotonin to Endurance Training," *Journal of Applied Physiology,* 46 (1979): 19–23.

4. Robert E. Dustman, et al., "Aerobic Exercise Training and Improved Neuropsychological Function of Older Individuals," *Neurobiology of Aging,* Fayetteville, NY (Spring 1984): 34–42.

5. Caryle H. Folkins, and Wesley Sime, "Physical Fitness Training and Mental Health," *American Psychologist* (April 1981): 373–89.

6. R. J. Young, Ph.D., "The Effect of Regular Exercise on Cognitive Functioning and Personality," *British Journal of Sports Medicine,* 13 (1979): 110–17.

7. Patricia Del Rey, "Effects of Contextual Interference of the Memory of Older Females in Differing Levels of Physical Activity," *Perceptual and Motor Skills,* 6(2)(April 10, 1983): 171–80.

8. M. Elsayed, et al., "Intellectual Difference of Adult Men Related to Age and Physical Fitness Before and After an Exercise Program," *Journal of Gerontology* (May 1980) 383–87.

9. Daniel B. Carr, et al., "Physical Conditioning Facilitates the Exercise-Induced Secretion of Beta-Endorphin and Beta-Lipotropin in Women," *The New England Journal of Medicine,* 305(10) (Sept. 3, 1981): 560–63.

10. David Sinyor, et al., "Aerobic Fitness Level and Reactivity to Psychosocial Stress, Physiological, Biochemical and Subjective Measure," *Psychosomatic Medicine,* 45 (June 1983): 205–14.

11. "Jogging for Mental Health: Believers and Skeptics Collide," *Psychiatric News* (Sept. 16, 1983): 38–39.

12. Sharla Lichtman, and Ernest Poser, "The Effects of Exercise on Mood and Cognitive Functioning," *Journal of Psychosomatic Research* 27 (11) (1983): 43–52.

13. Richard Powell, "Techniques for Differentiating Cortical Hemispheric Activity Following Exercise," *Perceptual and Motor Skills* 54 (June 1982): 923–32.

14. Erik Peper, Ph.D., Center for Interdisciplinary Science, San Francisco State University, "The Treatment of Asthma: Combining Biofeedback, Family Therapy and Self-Regulation," paper presented at the Society for Biofeedback of America meeting, New Orleans, La., April 14, 1985.

15. Ruth Winter, "Fitness Benefits," *Harper's Bazaar,* August 1982, 148–50.

5. Fine-Tuning Your Brain with Music

1. Charles Marwick, "Leaving Concert Hall for Clinic, Therapists Now Test Music's 'Charms.'" *Journal of the American Medical Association,* January 24/31, 1996, vol 275, no. 4, pp. 267–68.

2. M. H. Thaut et al., "Rhythmic Auditory Stimulation in Gait Training for Parkinson's Disease Patients," *Movement Disorders* 1996 March, 11 (2): 193–200.

3. "New Insights Explain Movement Control by the Brain," *News and Features,* National Institutes of Health, April 1984.

4. Ruth Winter, "Music: The New Active Sport," *Self,* May 1984, p. 175.

5. Manfred Schroeder, Ph.D., researcher, AT&T Bell Laboratories, "Monoaural Phase Effects in Masking with Multicomponent Signals," Symptoisum on Hearing-Physiological Bases and Psychophysics, Bad Nauheim, West Germany, April 5–9, 1983.

6. Rachel Nowak, "Brain Center Linked to Perfect Pitch," *Science,* vol. 267, 3 February 1995, p. 616.

7. "Music's Mystery: How It Works in the Brain," *New York Times,* May 16, 1995, p. C1.

8. I. Peretz, M. Tramo, et al., "Functional Dissociation Following Bilateral Lesions of Auditory Cortex," *Brain,* 1994, Dec., 117 (pt 6): 1283–301.

9. Music's Mystery: How It Works in the Brain, *New York Times,* May 16, 1995, C1.

10. R. J. Zatorre, A. C. Evans, E. Meyer, "Neural Mechanisms Underlying Melodic Perception and Memory for Pitch," *Journal of Neuroscience,* 1994 Apr., 14(4): 1908–19.

11. Winter, op. cit.

12. M. G. Safranek, "Effect of Auditory Rhythms on Muscle Activity," *Physical Therapy,* 62(2) February 1982: 161–68.

13. Winter, op. cit.

14. Ibid.

15. Avram Goldstein, "Thrills in Response to Music and Other Stimuli," *Physiological Psychology* 1980 vol. 8 (1), 126 29.

16. Kathy Brunet, "Rutgers-Newark Researcher Demonstrates That Listening to Music Has a Measurable Effect on Reducing Physical Pain," Rutgers news release, November 17, 1992.

17. Marwick, op. cit.

18. "Project Will Test Theory of Music and Brain Function," University of California, Irvine, news release, January 8, 1993.

19. "Babies Tune in Early to Music Psychologists Find," Stanford Story Source, Stanford News Service, June 1993.

20. "Study Shows Spatial IQ Test Scores Higher After Mozart," University of California at Irvine press release, Oct. 13, 1993.

21. Winter, op. cit.

22. "Scheming of Human Brain Helps Overcome Language Impairment," Stanford University Medical Center release, Feb. 8, 1984.

23. Winter, op. cit.

24. Trotter, R. J., "The Sight of Music Read in the Face," *Psychology Today*, March 18, 1985.

25. Winter, op. cit.

26. Ibid.

27. Ibid.

6. How to Improve Your Memory

1. Marian Cleeves Diamond, "The Aging Rat Forebrain: Male-Female Left-Right: Environment and Lipofuscin" in *Aging of the Brain*, ed. D. Samuel, et al. (New York: Raven Press, 1983).

2. J. W. Newcomer, S. Craft, et al., "Glucocorticoid-Induced Impairment in Declarative Memory Performance in Adults," *Journal of Neuroscience* 1994 Apr. 14(4): 2047–53.

3. Max V. Mathews, David E. Meyer, and Saul Sternberg, "Exploring the Speed of Mental Processes," Bell Telephone Laboratories *Record*, Murray Hill, NJ, March 1975, 150–56.

4. W. Penfield, and B. Milner, "Memory Deficit Produced by Bilateral Lesions of the Hippocampal Zone," *American Medical Association Archives of Neurology and Psychiatry*, 7 (1958): 475.

5. Anders K. Ericsoon, et al., "Aquisition of a Memory Skill," *Science*, 208 (June 6, 1980): 1181–182.

7. Expand Your Capacity to Learn

1. Nicholas Wade, "Method and Madness," *New York Times Magazine*, Feb. 22, 1994, p. 24.
2. Bill Cannon, "All the Rage," *Biomedical Inquiry*, University of Texas, Fall 1996 pp. 10–15.
3. Warner K. Schaie, ed., *Longitudinal Studies of Adult Psychological Development* (New York: Guilford Press, 1983).
4. Ruth Winter, "Are You As Smart As You Once Were?" *Register and Tribune Syndicate*, Des Moines, Iowa, Feb. 7, 1982.
5. Raymond B. Cattell, *Abilities: Their Structure, Growth, and Action* (Boston: Houghton Mifflin, 1971).
6. Winter, op. cit.
7. Gregory Clark, "Cell Biological Analysis of Associative and Non-Associative Learning," paper presented at the Annual Meeting of the American Association for the Advancement of Science, New York, May 26, 1984: University of Illinois at Urbana *News Feature*, Dec. 18, 1980. Eric Kandel, and James Schwartz, "Molecular Biology of Learning: Modulation of Neurotransmitter Release," *Science*, 218 (Oct. 29, 1982): 433–42.
8. Special Report on Aging, U.S. Department of Health, NIH Pub. No. 80-1907, Feb. 1980.
9. University of Illinois at Urbana-Champaign News Bureau Report, April 1996.
10. William Dember, and Joel Warm, "Effects of Fragrances on Performance and Mood in a Sustained-Attention Task," paper presented at the American Association for the Advancement of Science Annual Meeting, Washington, D.C., February 14, 1991.
11. D. Klein, R. J. Zatorre, B. Milner, E. Meyr, A. C. Evans, "Left Putaminal Activation When Speaking a Second Language: Evidence from Pet" *Neuroreport* 1994 Nov. 21;5 (17): 2295–7.
12. "A Window to the Brain: Where Linguistics and the Brain Sciences Meet, Insights Flow in Both Directions," *Mosaic*, 7 (March–April 1976) 14–25.
13. William Dement, M.D., presentation, news conference on insomnia, New York, NY 1996.
14. M. H. Kryger, "Is Society Sleep Deprived," *Sleep*, 1995, 18(10): 901; Y. Harrison and J. A. Home, "Should We Be Taking More Sleep," *Sleep*, 1995, 18(10):901–907; M. H. Sonnet and D. L. Arand, "We Are Chronically Sleep Deprived," *Sleep*, 1995, 18(10):908.
15. Avi Karni, et al., "Dependence on REM Sleep of Overnight Improvement of a Perceptual Skill," *Science* Vol 265, July 29, 1994 p 679–81;

Barinaga, Marcia, "To Sleep, Perchance to Learn? New Studies Say Yes," *Science* Vol. 265, 29 July 1994, p. 603.

8. Free Your Creativity

1. Beth Ann Krier, "Engineers Work on Developing the 'Fun Sides' of Their Brains," *Los Angeles Times*, March 16, 1984, p. 16.
2. "Visionaries and Madmen: Are Creativity and Schizophrenia Linked?" University of California Clip Sheet, University of California, Oct. 1, 1977.
3. Ibid.
4. Frederic Flach, M.D., "A Reappraisal of the Creative Process," *Psychiatric Annals*, March 1978, vol. 8, no. 3, pp. 11–22; Frederic Flach, interview with author, April 27, 1975.
5. Dr. Jan Ehrenwald, "The Anatomy of Genius: Split Brains and Global Minds," Human Science Press in 1984.
6. Beth Krier, op. cit.
7. Jerre Levy, and M. Reid, "Variations in Writing Posture and Cerebral Organization," *Science,* 194 (1976): 337–39.
8. Frederic Flach, interview with author, New York, April 27, 1975.
9. Morris Stein, Ph.D., "Methods to Stimulate Creative Thinking," *Psychiatric Annals,* 8(3) (March 1978) 65.
10. Bernice Neugarten, and D. Gutman, *Age-Sex Roles and Personality in Middle Age: A Thematic Apperception Study in Middle Age and Aging* (Chicago: Chicago University Press, 1975).

9. Food and Supplements to Fuel Your Brain

1. Sheryl Grady, et al., "Neuropsychological Function and Regional Cerebral Glucose Utilization in Health, Aging and Dementia," paper presented at the Society for Neuroscience meeting, Boston, Mass., Nov. 10, 1983.
2. J. A. Pulsinelli, et al., "Diabetes Mellitus," *Journal of the American Medical Association,* 74 (1983): 540–44.
3. *Good Housekeeping,* February 1984, p. 222.
4. Ibid.
5. Arthur Winter, M.D. and Ruth Winter, M.S., *Eat Right Be Bright,* (New York: St. Martin's Press, 1988).
6. Robert Butler, *Nutrition in the 1980s: Constraints on Our Knowledge* (New York: Alan Liss, Inc., 1981).

7. Alan F. Sved, "Precursor Control of the Functions of Monoaminergic Neurons," *Nutrition and the Brain* (vol. 6), eds. R. J. Wurtman and J. S. Wurtman (New York: Raven Press, 1983).

8. John Fernstrom, et al., "Diurnal Variations in Plasma Concentrations of Tryptophan, Tyrosine, and Other Neutral Amino Acids: Effects of Dietary Protein Intake," *American Journal of Clinical Nutrition* 32 (September 1979): 1912–22.

9. Carol Ballentine, "The Essential Guide to Amino Acids," *FDA Consumer*, 19 (7): 23–24.

10. A. J. Gelenberg, et al., "Tyrosine for the Treatment of Depression," *American Journal of Psychiatric Research*, 17 (2) (1982–83): 175–80.

11. Timothy Maher, "Natural Food Constituents and Food Additives: The Pharmacologic Connection," *Journal of Allergy and Clinical Immunology* 79 (3): 413–21.

12. S. Seltzer, et al., "The Effects of Dietary Tryptophan on Chronic Maxillofacial Pain and Experimental Pain Tolerance," *Journal of Psychiatric Research* 17:181–6, 1982–83; T. B. King, "Pain and Tryptophan," *Journal of Neurosurgery* 53(1): 44–55, 1980.

13. B. P. Maurizi, "The Therapeutic Potential for Tryptophan and Melatonin: Possible Roles in Depression, Sleep, Alzheimer's Disease, and Abnormal Aging," *Medical Hypotheses*, (1990) 32: 233–42.

14. "Clinical Spectrum of Eosinophilia-Myalgia Syndrome," *Morbidity and Mortality Weekly Report*, Centers for Disease Control, February 16, 1990, vol. 39, no. 6, pp. 1–3.

15. John Fernstrom, "Acute and Chronic Effects of Protein and Carbohydrate Ingestion on Brain Tryptophan Levels and Serotonin Synthesis," *Nutrition Reviews Supplement* 44 (May 1986): 25–35.

16. E. H. Reynolds, "Folic Acid, S-Adenosyl Methionine and Affective Disorders," *Psychological Medicine*, 13 (4): 705–10.

17. Arthur Winter, M.D., "New Treatment for Multiple Sclerosis," *Neurological and Orthopedic Journal of Medicine and Surgery* 5 (April 1984): 39–43.

18. *National Institute of Mental Health Science Reporter*, March 1984, S-3.

19. Paul Teychenne, *Questions and Answers About Parkinson's Disease and It's Treatment* (East Hanover, N.J.: Sandoz Pharmaceutical Co., 1985).

20. J. H. Pincus, and K. M. Barry, "Dietary Methods for Reducing Fluctuations in Parkinson's Disease," *Yale Journal of Biological Medicine* 60 (2): 133–37.

21. Ibid.

22. "Change in Diet for Victims of Parkinson's Disease," *Tufts University Diet and Nutrition Letter* 5(4).

23. Ruth Winter, M.S., *Super Soy: The Miracle Bean,* (New York: Crown Publishers, 1996.)

24. "Potato Dilemma: To Bake or Fry?" *Science News,* Feb. 4, 1984, 125.

25. Michael Trulson, paper presented to the 95th Annual Meeting of the American Psychological Association, New York, 31 August 1987.

26. Herman Baker, personal communication with authors, Feb. 13, 1987.

27. B. Regland, et al., "Vitamin B-12–Induced Reduction of Platelet Monoamine Oxidase Activity in Patients with Dementia and Pernicious Anemia," *European Arch of Psychiatry Clinical Neuroscience* 1991; 240(4–5) 288–91.

28. T. Ikeda, et al., "Treatment of Alzheimer-Type Dementia with Intravenous Mecobalamin," *Clinical Therapeutics* 1992 May June; 14 (3): 426–37.

29. L. Parnetti, et al., "Platelet MAO-B Activity and Vitamin B-12 in Old Age Dementias," *Molecular Chemistry and Neuropathology* 1992 Feb.–Apr.; 16(1–2): 23–32.

30. "Even Mild Lack of B-12 Could Hurt Seniors," Tufts University *Diet and Nutrition Letter,* vol. 9, no. 11, January 1992, pg. 1.

31. D. J. Pine, and E. D. Soria, "Myths About Vitamin B-12 Deficiency," *Southern Medical Journal* 1991 Dec.; 84(12): 1475–81.

32. J. Dommisse, "Subtle Vitamin B-12 Deficiency and Psychiatry: A Largely Unnoticed but Devastating Relationship," review article, *Medical Hypotheses* 1991 Feb.; 34 (2): 131–40.

33. Robert Russell, *Agricultural Research Services Research Briefs,* April–June 1991, p. 5.

34. T. R. Guilarte, "Vitamin B-6 and Cognitive Development: Recent Research Findings from Human and Animal Studies," *Nutrition Review* 1993 July 51 (7): 193–8.

35. S.K. Gaby, "Vitamin B-6," *Vitamin Intake and Health: A Scientific Review,* Marcel Dekker, New York, 1991, pp. 163–74.

36. J.R. Saltzman, K.V. Kowdley, M.C. Pedrosa, T. Sepe, et al., "Bacterial Overgrowth Without Clinical Malabsorption in Elderly Hypochlorhydric Subjects," *Gastroenterology* 1994 March; 106 (3): 615–23.

37. Richard Rivlin, "Riboflavin," *Present Knowledge in Nutrition,* 5th ed., 318–31.

38. E. H. Reynolds, "Interictal Psychiatric Disorders: Neurochemical Aspects," *Advanced Neurology* 1991; 55:47–58.

39. M.I. Boetz, "Neurological Correlates of Folic Acid Deficiency: Facts and Hypotheses," *Folic Acid in Neurology, Psychiatry, and Internal Medicine*, New York, Raven Press, 1979: 435–61.

40. S. Goldstein, "The Biology of Aging: Looking to Defuse the Genetic Time Bomb," *Geriatrics* 1993 Sep; 48 (9A): 76–82.

41. Warsama J. Jama, "Beta Carotene Said to Protect Against Cognitive Impairment," American Journal of Epidemiology, 1996; 144:275–80; and *Medical Tribune*, September 5, 1996.

42. P.A. Lewitt, "Neuroprotection by Antioxidant Strategies in Parkinson's Disease," *European Neurology* 1993; 33 Suppl 1: 24–30; S. Fahn, "A Pilot Trial of High-Dose Alpha-Tocopherol and Ascorbate in Early Parkinson's Disease," *Annals of Neurology*, 1992; 32 Suppl:S128–32.

43. D. S. Collier, et al., "Parkinsonism Treatment: Part III-Update," *Annals of Pharmacotherapy* 1992 Fe.; 26(2): 227–33.

44. L. Bischot, et al., "Vitamin E in Extrapyramidal Disorders," *Pharmacology World Science* 1993 Aug 20; 15 (4): 146–50.

45. Shantilal N. Shah, Ph.D., and Ronald C. Johnson, Ph.D., "Antioxidant Vitamins A and E Status of Down's Syndrome Subjects" *Nutrition Research*, vol. 9, pp. 705–15, 1989.

46. G. Milner, "Ascorbic Acid in Chronic Psychiatric Patients—A Controlled Trial," *British Journal of Psychiatry* 109 (1963): 294–99; N. Subramanian, "On the Brain: Ascorbic Acid and Its Importance in the Metabolism of Biogenic Amines," *Life Sciences* 20 (9); 1479–84.

47. D. Benton, and G. Roberts, "Effect of Vitamin and Mineral Supplementation on Intelligence of a Sample of School Children," *Lancet* 1: (1988) 140–43.

48. Robert Young, and John Blass, "Nutrition and the Aged," *Sourcebook on Food and Nutrition*, 3rd ed., Chicago, Il., Marquis, 1982, pp. 368–72.

49. Kaymar Arasteh, "Elevation of Mood with Calcium and Vitamin D," paper presented at the 95th Annual Meeting of the American Psychological Assn., New York, 31 August 1987.

50. E. Pollitt, and R. L. Leiberl, "Iron Deficiency and Behavior," *Journal of Pediatrics*, 88 (3) (1976): 372–81.

51. Ibid.

52. "Zinc Deficiency Retards Brain Development in Rat Studies," U.S. Dept. of Agriculture Report, Washington D.C., Nov. 10, 1983.

53. Frank G. Lawlis, Ph.D., et al., "Impacts of Food and Chemicals on Behavior," paper presented at the American Psychological Association meeting, Toronto, Canada, Aug. 27, 1984.

54. David Margulies, Beatriz Moisset, Michael Lewis, Hauo Shibiga,

and Candace Pert, "Beta Endorphin Is Associated with Overeating in Genetically Obese Mice and Rats," *Science,* 202 (Dec. 1, 1978): 89–99.

55. National Institute of Child Health and Human Development, "NICHD Guide for Researchers" Bethesda, MD., 1987.

10. Protecting Your Brain Against Potentially Harmful Chemicals

1. W. C. Abraham, Ph.D., et al., "Chronic Ethanol Effects on Sympathetic Function and Distribution in the Rat Hippocampus," paper presented at the Tenth Annual Meeting of the Society For Neuroscience, Cincinnati, Ohio, Nov. 1980.

2. Bernice Porjesz, and Henri Begleiter, "Evoked Brain Potential Differentiation Between Geriatric Subjects and Chronic Alcoholics with Brain Dysfunction," *Annals Neurology,* 32 (1982): 117–24.

3. I. Nylander, et al., "Differences Between Alcohol-Preferring and Alcohol-Avoiding Rats in the Prodynorphin and Proenkephalin Systems," *Alcohol Clinical Exp. Research* 1994 Oct.; 18(5): 1272–79; M. E. Charness, R. M. Safran, G. Perides, "Ethanol Inhibits Neural Cell-Cell adhesion," *Journal of Biochemistry* 1994 March 25; 269 (12): 9304–9; R. Ramanathan, et al., "Alcohol Inhibits Cell-Cell Adhesion Mediated by Human L1," *Journal of Cell Biology* 1996 April 133(2): 381–90.

4. "Alcohol Consumption and Intellectual Function in Elderly African-Americans," *Journal of the American Geriatrics Society* (1996; 44:1158–1165).

5. Peter Modica, "Light Alcohol Consumption May Boost Mental Function," *Medical Tribune News Service* Oct. 11, 1996.

6. Ibid.

7. E. Bernard Weiss, Ph.D., *Nutrition Update 1* (1983): 21–38; Charles Vorhees and R. E. Burcher, *Developmental Toxicology,* ed. K. Snell (London: Croom Helm, 1982).

8. Thomas Sobotka, Ph.D., "Revisions to the FDA's *Redbook* Guidelines for Toxicity Testing Neurotoxicity," *Critical Reviews in Food Science and Nutrition* 32 (2)(1992): 165–71.

9. J. W. Olney, "The Toxic Effects of Glutamate and Related Compounds," the Ophthalmic Communications Society, presented at the Symposium on Nutrition, Pharmacology, and Vision, sponsored by the Committee on Vision, National Research Council, National Academy of Sciences, Washington, D.C., Nov. 16–17, 1981.

10. Ibid.

11. Elaine E. Tseng, M.D., Malcolm Brock, M.D., Molly Lange, et al. "Excitatory Neurotoxins: Brain Damage May Be Reduced in Heart Surgery," paper presented at the American College of Surgeons' Annual Meeting, San Francisco, Calif., Oct. 8, 1996.

12. "Pharmacologic Treatments of Alzheimer's," *L'Année Géron-tologique; Facts and Research In Gerontology*, 1991, p. 57.

13. *FDA Backgrounder*, October 1991, Washington, D.C.

14. Ruth Winter, *A Consumer's Dictionary of Food Additives* (New York: Crown Publishers, 1994).

15. Ruth Winter, personal communication with author, March 14, 1990.

16. H. G. Pope, Jr., D. Yurgelun-Todd, "The Residual Cognitive Effects of Heavy Marijuana Use in College Students," *Journal of the American Medical Association*, 1996 Feb. 21; 275(7): 560–61.

17. P. A. Fried, "It's Easy to Throw the Baby Out with the Bath Water," *Life Sciences* 1995; 56 (23–24): 2159–68.

11. Chemicals for the Mind

1. Patric McGeer, professor emeritus, University of British Columbia, paper presented at the American Chemical Society Meeting, Chicago, Il, August 22, 1995.

2. M. X. Tang, D. Jacobs, et al., "Effects of Oestrogen During Menopause on Risk and Age at Onset of Alzheimer's Disease," *Lancet* 1996 Aug. 17; 348 (9025): 429–32; Joan Stephenson, Ph.D., "More Evidence Links NSAID, Estrogen Use with Reduced Alzheimer Risk," *Journal of the American Medical Association*, May 8, 1996, vol. 275, no. 18, pp. 1389–90; V. W. Henderson, Hill Paganni, et al., "Estrogen Replacement Therapy in Older Women: Comparison Between Alzheimer's Disease Cases and Nondemented Control Subjects," *Archives of Neurology* 1994, dep, 51 (9): 896–900.

3. Personal communication with author, August 19, 1996.

4. H. Fillit, "Future Therapeutic Developments of Estorgen Use," *Journal of Clinical Pharmacology*, 1995 Sep; 35 (9 Suppl): 25S–28S: Speech before St. Barnabas Medical Center's Medical Education Department meeting co-sponsored by Ayerst-Wyeth, June 5, 1996, West Orange, N.J.

5. Johns Hopkins Release, Baltimore, Md., June 14, 1996.

6. Lenore Launer, Ph.D., et al., "High Blood Pressure at Mid-Life May Lead to Cognitive Impairment," *Journal of the American Medical Association*, 1995, 274:1846–51.

7. Suzanne Craft, Ph.D., "Insulin May Play Key Role in Alzheimer's

Disease," paper presented at the International Neuropsychological Society Meeting, February 1995.

8. M. Calvani, et al., "Acetyl-L-Carnitine: An Anti-Aging Agent for the Treatment of Dementia," *Aging Brain and Dementia: New Trends in Diagnosis and Therapy*, 1990 Alan R. Liss, Inc., New York, pp. 603–22.

9. C. Missale, et al., "Nerve Growth Factor in the Anterior Pituitary Localization in Mammotroph Cells and Cosecretion with Prolactin by Dopamaine Regulated Mechanism," Proceedings of the National Academy of Sciences, USA, 1996 April 30;93(9):4240–5; K.S. Chen, et al., "Synaptic Loss in Cognitively Impaired Aged Rats Is Ameliorated by Chronic Human Nerve Growth Factor Infusion," *Neuroscience* 1995 Sep, 68 (1):19–27; J. D. Cooper, et al., "Reduced Transport of Nerve Growth Factor by Cholinergic Neurons and Down-Regulated TrkA Expression in the Medial Septum of Aged Rats," *Neuroscience* 1994 Oct, 62(3):625–9; K. Ohnishi, et al., "Age-Related Decrease of Nerve Growth Factor-like Immunoreactivity in the Basal Forebrain of Senescence-Accelerated Mice," *Acta Neuropathology*, 1995, 90 (1):11–16.

10. A.L. Markowska, D. Price, V. S. Koliatrsos, "Selective Effects of Nerve Growth Factor on Spatial Recent Memory as Assessed by a Delayed Nonmatching-to-Position Task in the Water Maze," *Journal of Neuroscience* 1996 May 15, 16 (10):3541–8.

11. X.U. Chang, Ph.D., Chinese Academy of Sciences, "Synthesis of Huperrine A Analoguou and Their Inhibitory Activities of Acetylcholinesterase," paper presented at the 206th American Chemical Society Meeting, Chicago, Il, Aug. 25, 1993.

12. D. C. Dorman, et al., "Effects of an Extract of Gingko Biloba on Bromethalin-Induced Cerebral Lipid Peroxidation and Edema in Rats," *American Journal of Veterinary Research*, 1992 Jan, 53 (1):138–42.

13. Alan Kozikowski, "An Improved Synthetic Route to Huperzine A: New Analogues and Their Inhibition of Acetylcholinesterase," paper presented at the 206th American Chemical Society Meeting, Chicago, Il, Aug. 25, 1993.

12. Stop Stress from Short-Circuiting Your Brain

1. Robert Sapolsky, "Why Stress Is Bad for Your Brain," *Science*, vol. 273, Aug. 9, 1996.749–50.

2. Troell Jensen, M.D. et al., "Cerebral Atrophy in Young Torture Victims," *New England Journal of Medicine* 307 (21)(Nov. 18, 1982): 1341.

3. Richard S. Lazarus, "A Cognitive Oriented Psychologist Looks at Biofeedback," *American Psychologist* 30 (1975): 553–561.

4. W. Jiang, J. Blumenthal, et al., "Mental Stress-Induced Myocardial Ischemia and Cardiac Events," *Journal of the American Medical Association* 1966; 275 (21):1651–6; "Study Hints Mental, Not Physical Stress, Is Bigger Heart Problem," *New York Times*, June 6, 1996, p. C2.

5. Mary Asterita, Ph.D., Indiana University School of Medicine, paper presented at the Biofeedback Society of American meeting, New Orleans, April 13, 1985.

6. David Skuse, et al., "New Stress-Related Syndrome of Growth Failure and Hyperphagia in Children, Associated with Reversibility of Growth-Hormone Insufficiency," *Lancet*, 1996; 348: 353–58.

7. K.J. Helsing, et al., "Causes of Death in Widowed Population," *American Journal of Epidemiology*, 116 (3) (September 1982): 524–32.

8. Ester Fride, Martha Weinstock, and H. Gavis, paper presented at the Society for Neuroscience meeting, Boston, Ma., Nov. 8, 1983.

9. *Special Report on Aging*, U.S. Department of Health, NIH No. 80-2135, August 1980.

10. Bruce McEwen, Ph.D., *Rockefeller University Research Profile*, Spring 1984.

11. Donald G. Payan, M.D., University of California, San Francisco, "Substance P," paper presented at the American Association for the Advancement of Science meeting, Los Angeles, Ca, May 30, 1985.

12. *Psychiatric News*, April 5, 1985.

13. Edgar Wilson, M.D. and Carol Schneider, Ph.D., of the University of Colorado, paper on pain presented at the Biofeedback Society of America meeting, April 16, 1985.

14. Arthur Winter, M.D., *Surgical Control of Behavior*, Springfield, IL: Charles Thomas Publishers, 1971.

15. Sam Rosenfeld, "Conversations Between Heart and Brain," U.S. Department of Health, No. 017-024000764-1, Nov. 1977.

16. *Cardiovascular Research Report*, American Heart Association, Summer 1982.

17. Neal Miller, Ph.D., Rockefeller University, New York, "Some Professional and Scientific Problems and Opportunities for Biofeedback," paper presented at Biofeedback Society of America meeting, New Orleans, La., April 14, 1985.

18. Albert Freedman, Ph.D., et al., Lafayette Clinic and Wayne State University, "Beta-Adrenergic Vasodilating Mechanism in Temperature Biofeedback," paper presented at the Biofeedback Society of America meeting, New Orleans, La., April 13, 1985.

19. Aharon Shulimson, M.S., et al., "Diabetic Ulcers: The Effect of

Thermal Biofeedback on Healing," paper presented at the Biofeedback Society of America meeting, New Orleans, La., April 13, 1985.

20. Lilian Rosenbaum, Ph.D., "A Team Approach to Diabetes: Biofeedback-Family Therapist, Nurse, Educator, Dietitian and Diabetologist," paper presented at the Biofeedback Society of America meeting, New Orleans, La., April 14, 1985.

21. Robert Yolton, Ph.D., "Biofeedback Treatment of Strabismus," presented at the Biofeedback Society of America meeting, New Orleans, La., April 16, 1985.

22. James Raczynski, Ph.D., "Biofeedback Treatment of Elevated Intraocular Pressure," paper presented at the Biofeedback Society of America, New Orleans, La., April 16, 1985.

23. Marcella Fischer-Williams, M.D., et al., "Cerebral Palsy Treated with EMG Biofeedback Following Neurosurgery," paper presented at the Biofeedback Society of America meeting, New Orleans, La., April 13, 1985.

24. Miller, op. cit.

25. Michael Tansey, Ph.D., "Sensorimotor Rhythm Biofeedback Training: Its Clinical Application for Learning Disabilities," paper presented at the Biofeedback Society of America meeting, New Orleans, La., April 16, 1985.

26. Joel Lubar, Ph.D., and Judith Lubar, M.A., paper presented at the Biofeedback Society of America meeting, New Orleans, La., April 16, 1985.

27. Thomas S. Elder, Ph.D., University of New Orleans, paper presented at the Biofeedback Society of America meeting, New Orleans, La., April 14, 1985.

28. A.C. Chen, N., and Dworkin, S.F., University of Washington, paper presented at the American Pain Society meeting, San Diego, Ca., Sept. 9, 1979.

29. Ibid.

30. "Doctors Shun Hypnotism's Power to Ease Pain Say Stanford Experts," *Stanford University New Service* feature, Dec. 19, 1985.

31. R. B. Zjonc, "Emotion and Facial Efference: A Theory Reclaimed," *Science,* April 5, 1985.

32. Vega Militariu, psychologist, Culinary Institute of America, interview with author, Hyde Park, NY, Dec. 19, 1982.

33. T. O. Allen, N. T. Adler, J. H. Greenberg, M. Reivich, "Vaginocervial Stimulation Selectively Increases Metabolic Activity in the Rat Brain," *Science,* 211 (March 6, 1981).

14. Prepare for Tomorrow

1. "The Writing Life: It Takes Guts to Grow Old," *Writers Digest,* October 1983, 20–21.

2. Douglas Martin, "Patience? This Man Practically Invented It," *New York Times,* p. 1, section 3.

3. *New Woman,* October 1984.

4. Raymond Truex, and Malcolm Carpenter, *Human Neuroanatomy* (Baltimore, Md, William and Wilkins Co., 1964), 504.

5. Amos Arieli, Alexander Sterkin, Ad. Aertsen, and Amiram Grinvald, of the Weizman Institute of Science, Rehovot, Israel, paper presented the the Annual Meeting of the Society for Neuroscience, San Diego, Ca., Nov. 13, 1995.

Glossary

Words that appear in SMALL CAPITALS are also found in this glossary.

Acetylcholine. A NEUROTRANSMITTER that is released by nerve cells and acts on either other nerve cells or muscles and organs throughout the body. Acetylcholine is believed to be involved in memory function.

ACTH. Adrenocorticotropic hormone. A hormone controlled

Action potential. An electric burst that travels the length of the nerve cell and causes the release of a NEUROTRANSMITTER.

Adrenal gland. About the size of a grape, your two adrenal glands lie on top of each of your kidneys. Each adrenal gland has two parts. The first part is the medulla, which produces EPINEPHRINE and NOREPINEPHRINE, two hormones that play a part in controlling your heart rate and blood pressure. Signals from your brain stimulate production of these hormones. The second part is the adrenal cortex, which produces three groups of steroid hormones. The hormones in one group control the levels of various chemicals in your body. For example, they prevent the loss of too much sodium and water into the urine. Aldosterone is the most important hormone in this group. The hormones in the second group have a number of functions. One is to help convert carbohydrates, or starches, into energy-providing glycogen in your liver. Hydrocortisone is the main hormone in this group. The third group consists of the male hormone, androgen, and the female hormones, estrogen and progesterone.

Agonist. A drug, hormone, or NEUROTRANSMITTER that binds to a receptor site and triggers a response.

Alzheimer's disease. A deterioration of the brain with severe memory impairment.

Amino acids. Building blocks of PROTEINS and NEUROTRANSMITTERS.

Angiotensin. A powerful elevator of blood pressure, angiotensin is produced by the action of renin, an enzyme made in the kidneys. All of the components of the renin-angiotensin system have been found in the brain, and there are indications that they are part of the brain's mechanism for regulating blood pressure as well as for telling you when you should or should not drink fluids.

Antagonist. A drug, hormone, or NEUROTRANSMITTER that blocks a response from a receptor site.

Anticholinergic. The blocking of acetylcholine receptors, which results in the inhibition of nerve-impulse transmission.

Antioxidants. Substances, such as vitamin E, that help prevent damage from oxygen. *See* Free radicals.

ApoE4. A gene that produces the protein APOLIPOPROTEINE4. This particular form of the gene occurs more often in people with ALZHEIMER'S DISEASE than in the general population. Two other forms of the gene, apoE2 and apoE3 may protect against the disease.

ApolipoproteinE. A protein that carries cholesterol in blood and that appears to play some role in the brain.

Arteriosclerosis. Commonly known as "hardening of the arteries," arteriosclerosis includes a variety of conditions that cause the artery walls to thicken and lose elasticity.

Aspartic acid. A nonessential AMINO ACID.

Atherosclerosis. A form of arteriosclerosis. The inner layers of the artery walls are made thick and irregular by deposits of a fatty substance. The internal channel of the arteries becomes narrowed, reducing blood supply.

Autonomic nervous system. The division of the nervous system that regulates the involuntary vital functions, such as the activity of the heart and breathing.

Axon. The principal fiber of a nerve that transmits outgoing signals to other cells.

Beta amyloid. A protein found in dense deposits forming the core of NEURITIC PLAQUES.

Blood-brain barrier. A group of closely packed cells that keep some substances in the blood stream from entering the brain.

Calcium messenger system. As calcium ions increase in the cell, a specific receptor protein, calmodulin, interacts with other proteins to initiate cell responses, such as smooth muscle contraction. The calcium messenger system is believed to play a part in learning.

Capillaries. The smallest blood vessels, which route blood to individual cells.

CAT Scan. *See* Computerized axial tomography scan.

Catecholamines. A group of self-made chemicals, such as NEUROTRANSMITTERS and hormones, that can be made synthetically. Among the major catecholamines are DOPAMINE, NOREPINEPHRINE, and EPINEPHRINE. The catecholamines are involved in the regulation of blood pressure, heart rate, muscle tone, METABOLISM, and central nervous system function.

CCK. *See* Cholecystokinin.

Cell. The smallest unit of a living organism that is capable of functioning independently.

Cerebral cortex. The "thinking brain." The part of the brain most involved in learning, language, and reasoning.

Cerebral thrombosis. Formation of a blood clot in a vessel leading to the brain.

Cerebral vascular accident. Apoplexy, or stroke, an impeded blood supply to part of the brain.

Cholecystokinin. CCK. A hormone produced by the small intestine during the movement of food from the stomach into the intestine. CCK causes the contraction of the gall bladder, thus releasing bile into the small intestine, where the enzymes and other components of bile aid digestion. This hormone has also been found in the brain and may help to stop overeating.

Choline. Found in most animal tissues, either free or in combinations such as lecithin or ACETYLCHOLINE. Choline is being actively studied for its effects on brain neurotransmission and memory.

Cholinergic. Pertaining to ACETYLCHOLINE; the cholinergic system includes the nerve cells that contain acetylcholine and the nerves and proteins that are stimulated or activated by acetylcholine.

Cholinesterase. The enzyme that processes the NEUROTRANSMITTER ACETYLCHOLINE. There is a great deal of scientific interest in this enzyme, particularly in the study of ALZHEIMER'S DISEASE, because it is believed to be involved in poor memory function.

Chromosome. Humans have twenty-three pairs of chormosomes, one set from the mother, one from the father. Chromosomes contain DNA, sequences of which make up the GENES.

Clinical trial. A controlled study designed to test whether an intervention, such as a pharmaceutical, is safe and effective in humans.

Cognitive functions. All aspects of thinking, perceiving, and remembering.

Computerized axial tomography scan. CAT scan. A diagnostic test that uses a computer and X-rays to obtain a highly detailed picture of the brain.

Corticotropin-releasing factor. CRF. A NEUROTRANSMITTER involved in appetite and stress reactions.

CRF. *See* Corticotropin-releasing factor.

Cysteine. A nonessential AMINO ACID.

Cystine. A product of CYSTEINE, produced by oxidation and sometimes found in urine. Used to treat brittle nails.

Dementia. A broad term referring to a condition in which cognitive functions decline.

Dendrites. Spiderlike projections from the cell body that receive and send messages between nerve cells.

Diuretic. A drug that promotes the excretion of urine.

DNA. Deoxyribonucleic acid. A large double-stranded molecule within CHROMOSOMES; sequences of DNA make up GENES.

Dopamine. An intermediate in tyrosine metabolism and the precursor of NOREPINEPHRINE and EPINEPHRINE. Dopamine is involved in movement and mood.

Endorphins. Self-made tranquilizers and pain killers. Each endorphin is composed of a chain of AMINO ACIDS and acts on the nervous system to reduce pain.

Enkephalins. Self-made pain killers to which ENDORPHINS belong.

Epinephrine. Adrenaline. The major hormone of the ADRENAL GLAND, epinephrine increases heart rate and contractions, vasoconstriction or vasodilation, relaxation of the muscles in the lungs and of smooth muscles in the intestines, and the processing of sugar and fat.

Familial Alzheimer's disease. FAD. An early-onset form of Alzheimer's disease that appears to be inherited. In FAD several members of the same generation of a family are often affected.

Free radicals. Oxygen molecules with an unpaired electron that is highly reactive, combining readily with other molecules and sometimes causing damage to cells.

GABA. *See* Gamma-aminobutyric acid.

Gamma-aminobutyric acid. GABA. A compound, found in high concentrations in the brain, that functions as an inhibitory NEUROTRANSMITTER.

Gene. The biological unit of heredity, each gene is located at a definite position on a particular chromosome and is made up of a string of chemicals called gases, arranged in a certain sequence along the DNA molecule.

Gene mutation. An abnormality in the sequence of the bases of a GENE.

GHRH. *See* Growth hormone-releasing hormone.

Glucagon. A NEUROTRANSMITTER involved in glucose metabolism and hunger.

Glucose. Blood sugar and the main fuel for the brain.

Glucose metabolism. The process by which cells turn food into energy.

Glutamic acid. A nonessential AMINO ACID.

Glycine. A nonessential AMINO ACID, usually derived from gelatin.

Growth hormone-releasing hormone. GHRH. A hormone that stimulates the release of sex hormones and is being studied as a therapy for the wasting of old age and for AIDS patients.

Hippocampus. A structure deep in the brain involved in memory storage.

Hypoglycemia. Low blood sugar—the opposite of diabetes.

Hypothalamus. Brain control area involved in emotions, movement, and eating. Less than the size of a peanut and weighing a quarter of an ounce. This small area deep within the brain also oversees appetite, blood pressure, sexual behavior, sleep, and emotions, and sends orders to the PITUITARY GLAND.

LHRH. *See* Luteinizing hormone-releasing hormone.

Luteinizing hormone-releasing hormone. LHRH. A hormone that helps regulate sex hormones.

Metabolism. The normal process of turning food into energy.

MRI. Magnetic resonance imaging. A diagnostic tool that uses magnetic fields to generate a computer image of brain anatomy. MRI can be used to measure brain activity.

Monoamine. Containing one amine group.

Monoamine oxidase inhibitors. MAOI. A group of drugs that is used in the treatment of depression and that elevates the level of NEU-ROTRANSMITTERS by preventing their destruction by enzymes.

Monoaminergic. Nerve cells or fibers that transmit nerve impulses stimulated by the NEUROTRANSMITTERS DOPAMINE, NOREPINEPH-RINE, and SEROTONIN.

Nerve growth factor. NGF. A hormonelike substance that promotes repair of certain nerves.

Neuritic plaques. Deposits of amyloid mixed with fragments of dead and dying nerve cells.

Neurofibrillary tangles. Collections of twisted nerve cell fibers found in the cell bodies of nerves in ALZHEIMER'S DISEASE.

Neuron. The basic nerve cell of the central nervous system, containing a nucleus within the cell body, an AXON (a trunklike projection containing NEUROTRANSMITTERS and DENDRITES, spiderlike projections that send and receive messages).

Neuropeptide Y. A NEUROTRANSMITTER believed to cause carbohydrate craving.

Neuroscientist. A scientist who studies the brain and nerves.

Neurotensin. A peptide of thirteen amino acid derivatives that helps regulate blood sugar by its effects on a number of hormones, including insulin and GLUCAGON. It is also thought to play a part in pain suppression.

Neurotransmitters. Molecules that carry chemical messages between nerve cells. Neurotransmitters are released from nerve cells, diffuse across the minute distance between two nerve cells (synaptic cleft), and bind to a RECEPTOR at another nerve site.

Nerve growth factor. NGF. Believed to maintain and repair nerves in the brain.

NGF. *See* Nerve growth factor.

Norepinephrine. Noradrenaline, a hormone released by the ADRENAL GLAND possessing the ability to stimulate, as does EPINEPHRINE, but with minimal inhibitory effects. It has little effect on the lungs' smooth muscles and metabolic processes and differs from epinephrine in its effect on the heart and blood vessels.

Oxygen free radicals. Oxygen molecules with an unpaired electron that is highly reactive, combining readily with other molecules and sometimes causing damage to cells.

Oxytocin. A pituitary hormone that stimulates muscle contraction.

Parasympathetic nervous system. A group of nerve fibers that leave the brain and spinal cord and extend to nerve cell clusters (ganglia) at specific sites. From there they are distributed to blood vessels, glands, and other internal organs. Parasympathetic nerves are involved in heart rate, stimulating digestion, and contracting bronchioles in the lungs, pupils in the eyes, and the esophagus. The parasympathetic nervous system works in conjunction with the SYMPATHETIC NERVOUS SYSTEM.

Parathyroid gland. On the four corners of the THYROID GLAND, these pearl-sized glands produce parathyroid hormones, which work with calcitonin from the thyroid gland to control calcium in the blood. Calcium has a role not only in developing bones and teeth but also is involved in blood clotting and nerve and muscle function.

Peptidase. An enzyme that splits simple PEPTIDES or their derivatives.

Peptide. Two or more AMINO ACIDS combined in head-to-tail links. Generally larger than simple amino acids or the MONOAMINES, the largest peptides discovered thus far have forty-four amino acids. NEUROPEPTIDES signal the body's endocrine glands to balance salt and water. Opiate peptides can help control pain and anxiety. The peptides work with amino acids. A peptide is present at two ten-thousandths of its partner amino acid or one hundredth of a MONOAMINE.

PET scan. Positron emission tomography. An imaging technique that allows researchers to observe and measure brain activity by monitoring blood flow and concentration of substances, such as oxygen and glucose in the brain tissue.

Phospholipids. Molecules of fat in cell membranes.

Pituitary gland. The pea-sized gland situated at the base of the brain, once thought to be the master gland that gave "orders" to other glands. It is now known that the pituitary gland takes its orders from the HYPOTHALAMUS. The pituitary then sends out orders to the other glands in your body. The frontal lobe of the gland produces six hormones: growth hormone, which regulates growth; prolactin, which stimulates the breasts and has other functions that are as yet not clearly understood; and four other hormones that stimulate the thyroid, adrenals, ovaries in women, and testes in men. The back lobe of the pituitary produces two hormones: antidiurectic hormone, which acts on the kidneys and regulates urine output, and OXYTOCIN, which stimulates the contractions of the womb during childbirth.

Plaques. Patches or build up of junk in arteries or teeth.

Protease. An enzyme that splits a protein into smaller sections.

Protein. A molecule composed of amino acids arranged in a specific order that is determined by a GENE. Proteins include NEUROTRANSMITTERS, enzymes, and many other substances.

Receptor. A protein molecule, which may also be composed of fat and carbohydrate, that resides on the surface or in the nucleus of a cell and recognizes and binds a specific molecule of appropriate size, shape, and charge.

Receptor binding assay. A technique to determine the presence and amount of a drug, NEUROTRANSMITTER, or receptor in a biological system.

Releasing factors. Produced by the HYPOTHALAMUS and then sent to the PITUITARY GLAND where they cause the release of appropriate hormones. Among those that have been found are LUTEINIZING HORMONE-RELEASING HORMONE (LHRH), which affects the release of the sex hormones, and thyrotropin-releasing factor (TRF), which affects the release of the thyroid hormone. Both LHRH and TRF have behavioral effects. LHRH, for example, enhances mating behavior. TRF causes stimulation.

Restless legs syndrome. A sense of uneasiness, twitching, or restlessness that occurs in the legs after going to bed, frequently leading to insomnia. It may be relieved temporarily by walking about. Restless legs syndrome is thought to be caused by inadequate circulation or as a side effect of medication.

Serotonin. A NEUROTRANSMITTER thought to play a role in temperature regulation, mood, and sleep.

SPECT scan. Single photon emission computed tomography. An imaging technique that allows researchers to monitor blood flow to different parts of the brain.

Stroke. *See* Cerebral vascular accident.

Substance P. A NEUROTRANSMITTER believed to carry pain messages from the body to the brain and vice versa.

Sympathetic nervous system. Consists of nerve fibers that leave the brain and spinal cord, pass through the nerve cells clusters (ganglia), and are distributed to the heart, lungs, intestine, blood vessels, and sweat glands. In general, sympathetic nerves dilate the pupils, constrict small blood vessels, and increase heart rate. The system also involves circulating substances produced by the ADRENAL GLAND.

Synapse. The minute space between two neurons or between a neuron and an organ across which nerve impulses are chemically transmitted.

Thyroid gland. A butterfly-shaped gland located in the neck with a "wing" on either side of the windpipe. The gland produces thyroxine, which controls the rates of chemical reactions in the body. Generally, the more thyroxine, the faster the body works. Thyroxine needs iodine to function.

Vagus nerve. Literally the "wandering nerve," because it has such a wide distribution in the body, the vagus nerve connects the stomach to the brain and is involved in other autonomic functions, such as breathing and heart rate.

Index

Numbers in *italics* refer to illustrations

A and B list of stressors, 200–201
abstract reasoning
  and diet, 148, 152
  and music traiining, 82–83
acetylcholesterase, 172–73
  inhibitor, 179
acetylcholine, 146, 168, 177
  defined, 137–38, 231
  and estrogen, 174
  and memory, 171–73
acetyle-L-carnitine, 177
"acoustical perfume," 30
acoustical tile, 30
ACTH, 231
action potential, 231
acupuncture, 188
adenosine, 160
adhesives, 166–67
adjustment, 65
adrenal cortex, 231
adrenal glands, 64, 155, 182,
  239
  defined, 231
adrenal hormones, 184–85
adrenaline, 183. *See also*
  Epinephrine

aerobic activity, 61–70
  classes, 69
  list of exercises, 68–70
age
  and cerebellum, 53
  and changes in brain, 3, 4
  and creativity, 122, 134
  and diet, 141, 150–51, 153–55
  and fluid intelligence, 64
  and hearing, 26
  and increasing intelligence, 6
  and learning, 109–12
  and memory, 138
  and multivitamins, 156
  and neurotransmitters, 62
  preparing for, 209–11
  and reflex time, 62
  and taste, 38
"Age 60 rule," 4
agonist, 232
air conduction, 25
alcohol, 158, 161–62
aldosterone, 183, 231
alertness, 114
  and exercise, 65
  and smell exercise, 116–17

aluminum, 166
Alzheimer's disease, 8–9, 135, 138, 141
  defined, 232
  diagnosis, 204, 206–8
  and environment, 166
  and food additives, 164–65
  medications for, 172–79, 208
  and vitamin B-12, 149
  and vitamin E, 153–55
Amazing Maze exercise, 59
amenorrhea, 64
American Music Conference, 88
amino acids, 139–48
  competition, 143–44
  defined, 139–40, 232
  and diet, 144–48
  excitatory, 163–64
amnesia, 96
amygdala, 32–33
amyloid placques, 177
amyotrophic lateral sclerosis (Lou Gehrig's disease), 194
anabolic hormones, 168
anaerobic exercises, 69–70
anafranil, 168
anaphylactic shock, 164
androgen, 231
angiotensin, 183, 232
angular gyrus, 7
Another Finger Exercise, 57
antagonist, 232
antianxiety drugs, 208
antibiotics, 149, 168
anticholinergic, 232
antidepressants, 142, 168, 208
antidiuretic hormone (ADH), 183
antihistamines, 168
anti-inflammatories, 173
antioxidants, 138, 153–55, 232
anti-Parkinson medication, 208
antipsychotic drugs, 154
anvil (incus), 25

anxiety, 33, 65, 202, 208
apoE4, 232
apolipoprotein E, 232
appetite center, 159–60
Arasteh, Kaymar, 156
arginine, 142
aromatase, 175
art, 84, 113
  and right brain, 123, 125–29
arteriosclerosis, 232
aspartame, 143, 163–64, 165
aspartic acid, 232
aspirin, 173
associates, choosing, 132
association, 94
  Practice exercise, 97–98
asthma, 164
atenolol, 168
atherosclerosis, 232
atrophic gastritis, 176
atropine, 168
attention, 9, 114
  Getter exercise, 116
  Paying, exercise, 103
auditory center, 26
auditory nerves, 27, 72
autoimmune diseases, 186
automatic tasks, 2
autonomic nervous system
  defined, 26–27, 232
  and sound, 26, 73
axon, 5, 232, 236

Bach, 78
background "noise," 23
Backward Pickup exercise, 55
balance
  exercises, 54–56
  test, 52
Ball-and-String exercise, 20
bananas, 158
basal ganglia, 62
baseball, 60

basilar artery, 7
BEAM, 207
Beethoven, 78
belly breathing, 67
benign senile forgetfulness, 95
Berra, Yogi, 16, 52
beta amyloid, 177, 232
beta carotene, 153
beta-endorphins, 64, 159. *See also*
    Endorphins
Bharucha, Jashed, 77
bike riding, 69
biochemical changes, 1, 6
biofeedback
    computerized, 208
    do-your-own, 195
    and music, 79
    and pain, 195
    and paralyzed limbs, 50, *51*
    and stress control, 191–96
bipolar disorders, 169
bitter taste, 38, *39*
Blanket Roll exercise, 56
blocadren, 100
blood-brain barrier, 143–44, 233
blood-clotting factors, 184
blood flow, 1
    and caffeine, 159
    and estrogen, 174
    and sensory input, 17
    and smiling, 199
blood pressure
    and brain, 33, 175–76
    medication, 168
    and music, 26, 87
    and personality, 189–90
    and stress, 183, 184
Blumenthal, James, 182
body-movement exercises, 56–57
body temperature, 42
    exercises, 43
Bolino, Frank, 174
bookcases, 30

Book on-Head Routine, 54–55
bowling, 60
Brahms, 78
brain
    areas defined, 7
    and blood flow, 1
    and chemicals harmful to, 161–70
    and coordination and motor skills,
        46–60
    and creativity, 122–34
    and diet and nutrition, 135–60
    drugs beneficial to, 171–79
    injury, 7–8
    and learning, 1–3, 109–21
    left and right, 125–29
    lost function, reversibility, 49–51
    and memory, 90–108
    and movement, 47–50
    and music, 71–89
    and physical exercise, 61–70
    portion used, 6–7
    research, future of, 210–11
    and senses, 11–45
    and smell, 32–33
    and stress, 180–203
    and temperature, 42
    types of cells composing, 6
    weight, 4, 6
    working out, 6–10
    young vs. old, 3–4
brain-body connection, 183–85
brain breathing exercises, 66–70
brain cells
    and age, 4
    and memory, 90–91, 93
    and music, 26
    types, 6
brain map, 14, 50, 207
    and fingers and hand, 47–49
    and music, 78
    and quadriplegics, *51*
brain stem, 32
brain waves, 194

Breaking Things Into Chunks, 104
breathing, 66–67, 87
Breath Relaxer exercise, 67
Bremner, Douglas, 181
Broca's area, 7, 119
Buckholtz, Neil, 174
Buckner, Randy L., 1
B-vitamin complex, 137, 141, 148–53

cadence, 104
caffeine, 158–59, 178–79
calcium, 156, 237
calcium channel blockers, 177
calcium messenger system, 233
calculator, 106–7
capillaries, 233
carbohydrates, 141, 145
"cardiac psychosis," 12
carnitine, 177
Carpenter, Maclolm, 210
carpeting, 30
Carr, Daniel B., 64, 65
Carret, Philip L., 209–10
cataract surgery, 11
catecholamines, 233
categories, 104
CAT scans (computerized axial
    tomography)
    defined, 1, 207, 234
    and old vs. young brains, 3–4
    and stress, 181
Cattell, Raymond B., 110–11
cell, 233
central nervous system, 4–7
central sulcus, 7
cerebellum, 7, 52–54
    exercises, 55–60
    and music, 73–74
    and pain, 187
    and proprioceptors, 14
cerebral beriberi, 152
cerebral cortex, 174
    defined, 18, 233

and motor skills, 47–52
and senses, 18
and sound, 27
cerebral palsy, 193
cerebral thrombosis, 233
cerebral vascular accident, 233. See
    also Stroke
cerebrum, 52
challenges, setting new, 121
Chaplin, Charlie, 96
Charades, 57
Charging Your Mind exercise, 107
chemicals, harmful, 161–70
chemical signals, 5
children
    and environmental toxins, 167
    and food additives, 165–66
    and marijuana, 169
    and music, 83
    sexual abuse, 181
    and stress, 183–84
chlorpromazine, 152
cholecystokinin (CCK), 233
cholesterol, 184
choline, 137–39, 172
    defined, 233
choline acetyltransferase (CAT), 172
cholinergic system, 172, 233
cholinesterase, 172–73, 233–34
    inhibitors, 172–73
chromosome, 234
chronic pain, 187–88
cimetidine, 168
Circles and Squares exercises, 129
City Lights (film), 96
clinical trial, 234
clomipramine hydrochloride, 168
Cognex, 172
cognition
    defined, 9
    and music, 82–83
    and physical exercise, 62
cognitive functions, 234

cognitive rehabilitation, 7, 9, 208
cognitive stimulation, 208
Coin Stacker exercise, 57
color additives, 165–66
Common Senses exercise, 106
communication, 9, 201
computer, learning to use, 120
computerized biofeedback training, 208
concentration, 114
concentration camp victims, 181
Congreve, William, 81
Connor, James, 91
conscious, 128
consolidation, 94
cooking methods, 147
coordination, 53
  defined, 46–51
  exercises, 54–55
Corpus Callosum, 123
cortex, 6, 185
cortical nerve cells, 18
corticotropin-releasing factor (CRF), 204
cortisone, 168
Craft, Suzanne, 176
Creative Humor exercise, 130
creativity, 9, 122–34
  and emotional problems, 124–25
  exercises, 129–31
  ridding self of inhibitors to, 130–34
  and right brain, 123, 125–28
  and subconscious and preconscious, 128–29
Crick, Francis, 109
critical thinking skills, 113
cross-sectional technique, 110
crossword puzzles, 20, 43
crystallized intelligence, 111
cupping, 188
curtains, 30
curvature of the spine, 193–94

Cushing's syndrome, 182, 184
Cut It Out exercise 60
cyanocobalamin, 149
cycloserine, 168
cysteine, 234
cystein-S-sulfonic acid (CSS), 164
cystine, 234

dancing, 124
Darwin, Charles, 124
daydreaming, 133
decibels, 26, 29
decisions, 201, 206
DEET, 167
Dember, William, 117
dementia, 234
dendrites, 5, 91, 234, 236
depression, 65
  and creativity, 124–25
  and diet, 141, 149–51, 156
  drugs for, 179
  and memory, 96
  and stress, 181
  details, 201
diabetes, 136–37, 151, 176
  and biofeedback, 193
Diamond, Marian, 4, 6, 91
diclofenac sodium, 168
diencephalon, 95
diet and nutrition, 8, 135–60
  and amino acids, 139–48
  and blood sugar, 135–37
  and caffeine, 158–59
  and medications, 103
  and memory, 103, 137–38
  and pain, 157–58
  and vitamins and minerals, 148–57
digesitve system, 33
discipline, 133
dishwashers, 30
distancing self, 131
diuretics, 234

DNA, 234
Dobs, Adrian, 175
Doenges, Bessie, 122
Donaldson, Henry, 1
Don't Forget to Yawn exercise, 68
Don't Let Emotions Interfere
    exercise, 117
dopamine, 160, 233
    defined, 234
    and depression, 124–25
    and diet, 140–42, 146, 154
    and movement, 53, 62
    and Parkinson's disease, 144, 154
Down's syndrome, 154
D-phenylalanine, 143
drugs
    harmful, 167–70
    helpful, 171–79
    and memory, 103, 208
    and nose, 33
Duara, Ranjan, 3
Dudai, Yadin, 37
Duke, Linda, 113
Dyer, Sir Edward, 102

ear drum, 25
earplugs, 30
ears, 4, 6
    infections, 27
    ringing, 29
Eastern religious practice, 191
eating, 33, 62
education
    and Alzheimer's, 8–9
    and intelligence, 111
EEG
    and biofeedback, 192, 194
    exam, 207
    and quadriplegic, 51
    and hearing, 27
egg yolk, 138
Einstein, Albert, 109, 123
Eisenson, Jon, 86

Elder, S. Thomas, 194
electrical signals, 5, 33
electrical stimulation
    and pain, 188
    and paralyzed limbs, 50
electro-chemistry
    and brain-body connection, 183–85
    and memory storage, 95
electroshock therapy, 94
EMG (electromyographic activity),
    51, 192
emotion, 33, 62
    and creativity, 123–25
    and immune system, 124
    and memory, 96
    and music, 26, 78–85, 79–80
    and smell, 33, 34–35
    and unwanted sound, 30
Employ Your Sense of Smell for
    Alertness exercise, 116–17
end, starting at, 133
endocrine glands, 95
endorphins
    and appetite, 159, 160
    defined, 61, 234
    and exercise, 64
    and music, 80–81, 124
    and pain, 157–58, 186
    receptors, 162
    and sex, 203
    and touch, 41
    withdrawal, 187
enkephalins, 162, 234
environmental neurotoxins, 166–67
enzymes, 139
eosinophilia-myalgia syndrome
    (EMS), 142
epilepsy, 6, 95
epinephrine, 125, 231, 233
    and amino acids, 140
    and blood glucose, 136
    defined, 234
    and stress, 183

essential amino acids, 139, 142–43, 145
estrogen, 173–75, 231
  receptors, 174
ethmoid bone, 32
euphrasia, 168
European Community Scientific Committee for Food, 165
Evans, Dr. Denis, 162
evoked potentials, 27
excitatory amino acids (EAA), 163–65
excuses, 134, 203
exercise machines, 69. *See also* Physical exercise
exit list, 108
external auditory canal, 25
eyebright, 168
eyes and sight, 18–25
  and biofeedback, 193
  exercises, 18–22
  and nerves, 4, 6

lacedness, and music, 86–87
Face Identification exercise, 98
facial expression, 199
Familial Alzheimer's disease (FAD), 235
Fare, Gabriel, 134
Farming Your Brain, 133
fast pathway, 185
fatigue, and stress, 203
fatty acids, 160
fear reactions, 33
Feingold, Benjamin, 165–66
Fernald, Anne, 83
fetus
  and music, 78
  and stress, 184
fight-or-flight response, 27, 183, 185
Fillit, Howard, 174
Find That Beat exercise, 28–29

Finger Fun exercise, 60
fingering space, 15
fingers, and brain map, 47–49
fish, 172
Flach, Frederic F., 125, 128–29, 131
"flash bulb" memory, 92
flashlight exercises, 18–20
floor scrubbing, 69
fluid intelligence, 64, 111, *112*
fluorescent light, 24
focusing, 9
Fogel, Max, 110
folic acid, 148, 152–53, 156
food additives, 162–66
food allergy, 166
Food and Drug Administration (FDA), 163, 165, 172
free radicals, 153, 155, 235
free weights, 70
Freud, Sigmund, 96, 180
Friedman, Meyer, 189
frontal lobe, 7, *7*
  and auditory system, 27
  and taste and smell, 37
fruity odors, 33
frustrations, writing exercise, 133
Fuldheim, Dorothy, 210
Functional Electrical Stimulation (FES), 49–50

GABA (gamma-aminobutyric acid), 160, 235
galvanic skin resistance, 87
garage cleaning, 69
gardening, 69
Gardiner, Martin, 84
"gate" theory, 85
Gelenberg, Alan J., 140
gene, 235
  mutation, 235
Gengo, Fran, 168
Geriatrics, 153

Get Enought Sleep exercise,
    119–20
Ginkgo, 179
glia (glial cells), 6
glucagon, 235
glucocorticoid hormones, 180–81
glucose (blood sugar), 135–37, 152,
    155 defined, 235
  high vs. low, 136–37
  and insulin, 176
  and pain, 157–58
  and stress, 183
glue, 166–67
glutamate, 163–65
glutamic acid, 163–64, 235
glycine, 235
goals
  identifying, 202
  setting, 118
Goldstein, Avram, 80–81
Goldstein, S., 153
Goodwin, James S., 148
growth hormone, 184
growth hormone-releasing hormone
    (GHRH), 235
Gurvits, Tamara, 181
gustatory cortex, 37

hair cells, 25
hammer (malleus), 25
handball, 68
handedness tests, 127–28
hand-eye coordination, 55, 102
  and biofeedback, 194
  exercises, 58–60
hands, 46–48, 53
  dexterity exercises, 57
Hartmann, Ernest, 141
Hasan, Ziaul, 47
Have You Hugged Your Pillow
    Today? exercise, 41
headphones, 26

head trauma, 7
healing, and music, 73
hearing-oriented learner, 113–14
hearing sense, 16, 25–30
  exercises, 27–29
  on PET scan, 2
  protecting, 27
heart, and stress, 188–90
heart attack patients, 11–12
Hear the News exercise, 29
Hebb, Donald, 11
Heel to Knee test, 52
helper T cells, 186
high blood pressure, 191, 208
high-carbohydrate meals, 145–46
high-protein diet, 142, 143,
    146–47
Hilgard, Ernest, 197
Hilgard, Josephine, 197
hippocampus, 173–74, 176
  defined, 14, 235
  and memory storage, 91
  and stress, 180–85
hormones
  defined, 31
  and exercise, 64
  and light, 24
  and music, 73
  and smell, 33
  and stress, 183–84
Horn, John, 110–11
Hubel, David, 18
Human Anatomy (Truex and
    Carpenter), 210
hunger, 33
Huntington's chorea, 165
huperzine (Hup A), 179
hydergine, 208
hydrocortisone, 231
hyperactivity, 165, 166
hypnosis, 196–98
hypoglycemia, 136

hypothalamus, 62, 159–60, 174, 238
  defined, 33, 235
  and food additives, 164
  and pain, 185

Iacocca, Lee, 116
ibuprofen, 173
ice, for pain, 188
identifying stimuli, 27
IL-2, 174
illumination, 131
immune system, 124, 184, 186
Increase Your Arousal Level
  exercise, 116
incubation, 131
indomethacin, 173
ink blot test, 22
inner-eye pressure, 193
insect repellent, 167
insomnia, 141, 195
insulin, 139, 157, 160, 176
  receptors, 176
  and stress, 183
Integrating, 9
intelligence (intellect)
  and age, 6, 109–11
  defined, 90
  fluid vs. crystallized, 111
  and multivitamins, 156
  and music, 82–86
  post-injury, 8
intention, 104
iron, 157
isocarboxazid, 168

James, William, 104
Jefferson, Thomas, 100
"jet lag," 24
jigsaw puzzles, 20
jogging, 69, 74–75
*Journal of the American Medical
  Association,* 148

judgment, defering, 133–34
Jump Rope exercise, 68
Justice, Blair, 123

Karlsson, Jon, 124
Karni, Avi, 120
Katsch, Shelley, 28, 79–80
Kawas, Cladia, 8–9
Keats, John, 43
Keep a Diary exercise, 118
Keller, Helen, 16
Kitchen Timer exercise, 108
Kodaly method, 83–84, 84n
Koshland, Gail, 79
Kroll, Walter P., 49–50

Lacey, Beatrice, 189
Lacey, John, 189
Lacquer thinner, 167
Lancet, 157
Landfield, Philip, 184–85
language, 118–19, 123
  learning new, 118–19
  and music, 77
lateral sylvian sulcus, 7
Launer, Lenore J., 175–76
lavender, 37
Lawlis, Frank G., 157
Lazarus, Richard S., 181–82
L-dopa, 53
lead, 167
Learn a New Language exercise,
  118–19
learning, 109–21
  circuit for, 2
  defined, 90
  and diet, 156–57
  exercises, 114–21
  and heat, 42
  and intelligence, 111–12
  styles, 113–14
  two endeavors of, 109

learning disabilities, 194
Learning to Use Computer exercise, 120
lecithin, 137, 138, 146, 172
left and right brain hemispheres
   defined, 125–29, *126*
   and ear, 27
   tests for dominance, 127–28
left brain
   and exercise, 65
   and language, 77, 119
   and logic, 123
   and music, 76
   See also Right brain
left-faced people, 86
legumes, 145
leisure pursuits, 131–32
letter
   One-Page exercise, 130
   about stressor, 201
   To Yourself from Someone else
      exercise, 130
levodopa, 144
Levy, Jerre, 127, 128
Lewy, Alfred, 24
light exercises, 24–25
Lilly, John, 11
limbic system, 62
   defined, 32
   and music, 78
   and pain, 185, 186
   and stress, 185
Line Dancing, 56
Lip exercises, 38
List Memorization exercise, 98
Locked-In Syndrome, 7–8
longitudinal technique, 110
long-term memory, 93–94
Lopes, Carolos, 4
"losing" things, 95
Lou Gehrig's disease, 194
L-tryptophan supplements, 142
Lubar, Joel, 194

Lubar, Judith, 194
luteinizing hormone-releasing
   hormone (LHRH), 235, 238

McEwen, Bruce, 173
McNaughton, Bruce, 120
Make the Connections exercise, 58
Making Notes exercise, 107
Making Scent Associations exercise, 35–36
manic-depression, 124
marijuana, 169
Markowska, A. L., 178
Marplan, 168
martyr, avoid being, 201
massage, 41, 198–99
math
   and calculator, 106–7
   and music, 83–84
Mathews, Max, 93
Mattheson, Ella Tuttle, 209
Matthews, Karen A., 189
meditation, 198, 199
medulla, 7, 231
melanin, 140
melatonin, 24, 141
melody processing, 77
memory, 90–108
   and alcohol, 161
   and amygdala, 33
   chemicals to enhance, 171–79
   and choline, 137–38
   defined, 9, 90
   and diet, 152, 157
   and drugs, 168, 169
   improvement aids, 103–8
   and malnutrition, 148
   neurological exam for, 207–8
   process of, 91–96
   and professional help, 204–6
   and smell, 34–35
   and stress, 92–93
   storage, 93

training exercises, 96–103
  when to seek help for, 204–6
memory retrieval, 96
  exercise, 98, 100–102
memorization exercises, 98–100, 104
men, PET scans, 2
menopause, 173, 174
Mensa, 110
menstrual cycle, 183
mental rehearsal, 51
mental stress tests, 182
metabolism
  and aerobic exercises, 63
  defined, 3, 236
  and diet, 141
  and glucose, 235
  and light, 24
  and sensory input, 17
  and younger vs. older brains, 3
methionine, 142, 162
Meyer, David, 93
Michener, James, 210
migraine headaches, 169, 191, 195, 208
Miller, Neal, 192
minerals, 156–57
Mini-Mental State (MMS), 207
Mini-music vacation, 85
mistakes, 134
MK-801, 164
mnemonics, 97–103
monoamine oxidase (MAO), 149, 153–54, 236
monoamine oxidase inhibitors (MAOI), 149, 168, 236
monoaminergic, 236
mood
  and music, 28, 79
  and physical exercise, 64–65
  and scents, 36
  and vitamins, 156
motivation, 62
  and brain damage, 9

and cerebellum, 54
and mental exercises, 9
motor nerve, 5
motor skills, 46–52, 62, 72–74
  and age, 53
  and brain maps, 48–49
  restoration of, 5–6
movement-and-touch-oriented learners, 114
movements
  brain map of, *48*
  and oxygenation, 62–63
  relearning, 49–51, *51*
  symmetry, and pain, 187–88
Mozart, 84–85
MRA (magnetic resonance angiography), 208
MRI (magnetic resonance imaging), 180, 207, 236
MRS (magnetic resonance spectroscopy), 208
MSG (monosodium glutamate), 165
MSI (magnetic source imaging), 208
multiple sclerosis, 143
multiple vascular dementia, 174
multivitamins, 156, 208
muscles, and nerves, 4, 6
music, 71–89
  and babies, 78
  benefits of, 25–26, 71
  and emotion, 79–81
  and endorphins, 124
  exercises, 28–29
  how brain is affected by, 75–78
  and intellect, 82–84
  and mood, 28
  and pain, 81–82
  and right brain, 123
  studying to, 84–85
  workouts for brain, 85–89
musical imagery, 77–78
musical instrument, 74, 87–89

N-acetyltransferase, 138
naloxone, 80, 159, 178, 186
names, memorizing, 104
Naming Dog Breeds exercise,
    129
naproxen, 173
National Institute of Child Health
    and Human Development
    (NICHD), 160
National Institute of Mental Health,
    159
National Institute on Aging, 53,
    61–62, 111, 181, 184
National Institutes of Health (NIH),
    3, 4, 24, 120, 165, 175
neocortex, 32
nerve growth factor (NGF), 174,
    178, 236
nerves
    communication between, 5
    defined, 4
    and learning, 91
    and sense organs, 12–13
    and stereo vs. monaural music,
        75
Neugarten, Bernice, 134
neuritic plaques, 236
neuroanatomists, 32
neurobiology, 5–6
neurofibrillary tangles, 236
neuroimagery techniques, 50–51
neurological examination, 207–8
neurons (nerve cells)
    defined, 6, 236
    and diet, 140, 153
    and proteins, 37
    and signals, 5
neuropeptides, 237
neuropeptide Y, 236
neuroscientist, 3, 236
neurotensin, 236
neurotoxins
    and drugs, 167–70

    and estrogen, 174
    environmental, 166–67
    in food, 162–66
neurotransmitter chemicals, 231
    and amino acids, 139–40
    and creativity, 124
    defined, 236
    and diet and nutrition, 135,
        137–38, 144–45, 154, 160
    and memory, 95
    and oxygen levels, 62
    and pain, 186, 188
Newcomer, John, 92
New England Journal of Medicine,
    151
New Jersey Neurological Institute,
    50, 79, 191
News Program exercise, 29
New York Times, 122
niacin, 148
Nichols, Elaine, 78
Nightingale, Florence, 81
night shift, 24
no, learning to say, 203
nociceptors, 185
noise, 26–27, 29–30
nominal memory, 95
nondominant hand, 128
non-steroidal anti-inflammatory
    drugs (NSAIDS), 173
norepinephrine (noradrenaline),
    124, 231, 233
    defined, 62, 236–37
    and diet, 140, 141, 143, 146,
        160
    and exercise, 64
    and stress, 183
nose, 4
    pharmaceuticals through, 33
    touching test, 52
notes
    and creativity, 133
    and memory, 107

obesity, 159
Observation
  Practicing Powers of, 114–15
  Speeding up Powers of, 115–16
occipital lobe, 7
odor molecules, 31
odor sensory cells, 32
Oian Ceng Ta, 179
older people, 3–4
  education and, 8
  and memory problems, 96
  See also Age
olfactory bulb, 31–34
olfactory cells, 31
olfactory lobe, 32, 36
olfactory nerve, 7
Olney, John, 163
opiate receptors, 187
oral contraceptives, 168
organization, 9, 104
  information exercises, 118
  and learning, 114
  and memory, 104
osmone 1, 35
oval window, 25
overeating, 33, 159, 233
oxygen free radicals, 237
oxygen levels
  exercises to increase, 66–70
  and ginkgo, 179
  and neurotransmitters, 61–66
  and playing woodwinds, 87
  and smiling, 199
oxytocin, 183, 237, 238

pain
  control methods, 188
  diet and, 157–58
  music and, 81–82
  and stress, 185–88
  temperature feedback for, 195–96
painting, 69
panic disorders, 149

paradoxical breathing, 66
paralyzed limbs, 49–50, 208
Parasuraman, Raja, 117
parasympathetic nervous system, 237
parathyroid gland, 237
Parkinson's disease, 62, 144, 169
  and music, 72
  and Vitamin E, 153–54
Pat Yourself on the Head exercise, 57
Payan, Donald G., 186
pellagra, 141
Penfield, Wilder, 94–95
Pennebaker, James, 123–24
peptidase, 237
peptides, 139, 237
perceptual learning, 120
perfect pitch, 76
performance intelligence, 111
personality, 27, 189–90
pesticides, 167
Petersen, Steven E., 1
PET scanner (positron emission tomography), 2–3, 118
  defined, 1, 208, 237
  and exercising brain, 50–51
  and glucose, 135
  and memory, 91
phenelzine sulfate, 149
phenylalanine, 140, 143, 165
phenylketonuria (PKU), 143
Pherin Corporation, 33
pheromone, 31
phospholipids, 237
phosphorus, 37
physical exercises, 61–70
  and mood, 64–65
  as stress reliever, 202–3
Physionomie humaine (Waynbaum), 199
piano, 2, 52, 54, 73–75, 87–88
Picking Out Priorities exercise, 116
Pincus, Jonathan H., 144

pineal gland, 24
PIN numbers, 108
pitch, 76–77
Pitman, Roger, 181
pituitary gland, 64, 174, 184, 237–38
place, best for creativity, 133
placebo effect, 186
plants, and scents, 36–37
plaques, 238
Play Games exercises, 121
Playing with Blocks exercise, 131
Play Jacks exercise, 60
pleasure, 62
Pollitt, Ernesto, 137
post-traumatic stress disorder, 181
posture, 187
potassium, 158
potential, 27
practice, 48–49, 88
    and cerebellum, 52, 54
    PET scans and, 2–3
preconscious, 128–29
pregnancy, and stress, 184
premenstrual tension, 151
preparing self, and creativity, 131
priorities, 201
problem solving, 9, 123
    creativity steps for, 132–34
    and stress, 182
professional help, 204–6
progesterone, 231
proprioception sense, 13–14
protease, 238
    inhibitors, 177
protein, 136, 139
    defined, 238
    complete, 145
    importance of, in diet, 145
    and Parkinson's disease, 144
psycho-sclerosis, 122
Psychosocial Short Stature, 183–84
psychotherapy, 208
    and creativity, 128, 130–31

"Punnies" exercise, 130
Put the Squeeze On exercise, 60

quadriplegic, 51

racquet ball, 68
rage reactions, 33
Raichle, Marcus E., 2
Rauscher, Frances, 82, 84
Raymond, Gay, 79
Raynaud's disease, 179, 192–93, 208
RDAs, 151
reading, 24, 119
reasoning, 123
receptor, 238
receptor binding assay, 238
Red Dye No. 3, 165–66
Reeves, John, 68
reflex or reaction time, 61, 63
registration, 94
Rehearse, Rehearse, Rehearse
    exercise, 118
relaxation and stress control
        methods, 190–203
    biofeedback, 190–96
    hypnosis, 196–98
    massage, 198–99
    meditation, 198
    and smiling, 199
    what to do about, 199–203
    when to use, 203
releasing factors, 238
relevant information, 9
REM, 120
renin, 183, 232
repetition, 120
    and memory, 104
repression, 96
reproductive behavior, 62
respiration
    and music, 26, 87
    and smell, 34
Restaurant Guesser exercise, 39

restless legs syndrome, 238
reticular formation, 62
retina, 124, 164
retrograde amnesia, 94
review, 104
rhinencephalon, 32. *See also* Limbic
    system
rhythm, 25–26, 71–72, 75, 78–79
riboflavin, 148
rice, 145
right brain
    and creativity, 123, 125–29
    defined, *126*
    and hypnosis, 197
    and language, 77
    and music, 77, 79–80
    See also Left and right brain
    hemispheres
Robbins, Clive E., 82
role, don't play, 132
romantic mood, 29
Rorschach test, 22
Rosenman, Ray, 189
roses, 37
runner's high, 62
Russell, Robert, 150

S-adenosyl-L-methionine (SAM),
    142
Safranek, Monica Grenier, 79
Sagi, Dov, 120
salt (sodium), 158
salt taste, 38, *39*
same track, going over, 133
Sapolsky, Robert, 180, 182–83
Sargent, Thorton, 124
Saucy Saucer exercise, 57
saying aloud, and memory, 103
Scent Associations exercise, 35–36
scent memories, 32
Schaie, K. Warner, 110
Schiffman, Susan, 36
schizophrenia, 27, 124–25

Schlaug, Gotfried, 75–76
Schneider, Carol, 187
Schroeder, Manfred R., 75
Schul, Rina, 37
Science, 51, 96, 180
security, and creativity, 132
selective stimulation, 17–18
selegiline, 153–54
self-acceptance, 201
self-confidence, 65
self-esteem, and music, 80
self-knowledge, 123
Selye, Hans, 180, 183
senses
    developing, 16
    fatiguing, 17–19
    hearing, 25–30
    and memory, 104, 106
    and nerves, 4
    and neurons, 6
    organs, and brain, 12–13
    pleasure of, 43–45
    sight, 18–25
    smell, 30–37
    of space, 15
    taste, 37–39
    touch, 40–43
sensorimotor cortex, 194
sensory deprivation, 11–12
sensory experience, search for
    strong, 17
seromycine, 168
serotonin
    defined, 62, 238
    and diet, 140–42, 145
    and pain, 188
Set a List of Weekly and Daily Goals
    exercise, 118
Set New Challenges exercise, 121
sex
    and smell, 31, 33
    and stress, 203
Shatin, Leo, 28

Shaw, George Bernard, 134
Shaw, Gordon, 82
Sheline, Yvette, 181
Shelter, Donald, 85, 87
short-term memory, 93, 94, 96
Shrug It Off exercise, 56
shunting signals, 6
sight
  highly developed, 16
  exercises, 18–23
  See also eyes
sight-oriented learner, 113
silent zones, 49
Simon Sez, 56
singing, 6, 86, 87
sinus medication, 168
Sirigu, Angela, 51
skiing, 69
skin
  and biofeedback, 192
  and nerves, 4
  and sensory receptors, 40
  See also Touch
Skull Shining exercise, 67
sleep, 62
  and diet, 141
  and exercise, 65
  getting enough, 119–20
  and learning, 119–20
  and stress, 203
Slotnick, Burton, 37
slow pathway, 185
smell, 30–37
  and alertness, 116–17
  and behavior and memory, 34–36
  defined, 30–34
  exercises, 35–37
  and taste, 37
smiling exercise, 199
Smith, Karl U., 86
snail (cochlea), 25
solitude, and creativity, 132
solvents, 33

sound
  levels, 29
  paths to brain, 26–27
  unwanted, 30
sour taste, 38, 39
space/distance sense, 14–15
spatial intelligence, 84–85
spatial memory, 95, 120
SPECT scan (single photon
  emission computed
  tomography), 208, 238–39
speech, 2, 52
  retraining, and músic, 86
  therapy, 208
Speed Up Your Observation Powers
  exercise, 115–16
spinal cord, 4
Spring, Bonnie, 137
Square Dancing, 56
squash, 68
Stein, Morris, 131
Steinmetz, Helmuth, 75–76
Sternberg, Saul, 93
steroid hormones, 231
steroids, 168
Stimulate Your Olfactory Nerves
  exercise, 36
stirrup (stapes), 25
Stork Balance exercise, 55–56
strabismus, 193
stress, 180–203
  awareness, 190
  and body, 183–85
  and CAT levels, 172
  control methods, 190–203
  and diet, 141, 152, 155
  and exercise, 64
  and heart, 188–90
  and pain, 185–88
  steps to reduce, 200–203
  and writing about feelings, 124
stress hormones, 92–93, 183–85
stress-related aggression, 62

stretching exercises, 70
stroke, 7–8, 97, 137
    and music, 71–72, 77, 86
Strug, Kerri, 7
studying, 85
stutterers, 77
subconscious, 128–29
Substance P, 186, 239
Sudnow, David, 86, 87
sugar, in diet, 136–37. *See also*
    Glucose
sulfite, 164
sweet taste, 38, 39
swimming, 68
sympathetic nervous system, 239
synapses, 5, 91, 239
    and Alzheimer's disease, 8

Table-Topping exercise, 56
tacrine, 172, 208
Tagamet, 168
Take Notes from Print or Discussion
    exercise, 117
Take Your Temperature exercise, 43
Talk Like Animals exercise, 28
Tansey, Michael, 194
tardive dyskinesia, 154
taste, 16, 30, 37–39
    exercises, 38–39
tastebuds, 38, 39
television, 119
temperature
    Feedback, for pain control, 195
    Test Yourself exercise, 43
tempo, 25, 75, 78–79
temporal gyrus, 25
temporal lobe, 7, 76–77
tennis, 2, 54, 69
tenoretic, 168
tension, 190
testing
    and creativity, 131
    respiratory efficiency, 66–67

testosterone, 175, 183
thalamus, 25, 72, 73
    defined, 32
    and pain, 185
THA (tetrahydroaminoacridine), 172
Thaut, Michael H., 71, 72
thiamine, 148, 152, 156
thinking, 2
Think of a Song exercise, 86
thorazine, 152
thrill, 80–81
thyroid gland, 239
thyroid hormones, 140, 166, 183
thyrotropin-releasing factor (TRF),
    160, 238
Tillis, Mel, 77
time
    best for creativity, 133
    sense, 15–16
    zones, 24
timer, 108
timing sense, 55
timolide, 168
timolol maleate, 168
toluene, 167
tongue, 37–38
    map, 39
torture victims, 181
touch, sense of, 12, 16, 40–43
    defined, 40–41
    exercises, 41–43
Touch Identification exercise, 42
Touch Language, 41
Tramo, M. J., 76–77
tranylcypromine sulfate, 149
*Treatise on Neuroplasticity and
    Repair in the Central Nervous
    System* (WHO), 10
trigeminal nerve, 7, 33
    receptors, 33
Truex, Raymond, 210
Trulson, Michael, 147
tryptophan, 140–43, 145, 158

tumors, 95
tune, carrying, 86
Turn Down your Motor exercise, 133
Turn off the TV and Read exercise, 119
Tweezer Pickup exercise, 57
Type A and B personalities, 189–90
tyrosine, 140, 141, 143, 146

U.S. Congress, 4

vagus nerve, 239
valproate, 169
Van der Kilk, Bessel A., 187
vegetarian diet, 145
verbal intelligence, 111
vertebral artery, 7
Vietnam Head Injury Study, 8
violin playing, 87
Visual Scanning exercise, 20–21
Visual-Space Orientation exercise, 21
visual cortex, 18, 77
visual hallucinations, 124
visualization exercise, 102–3
Visual Scanning exercise, 20–21
Visual-Space Orientation exercise, 21
vitamin A, 153, 154–55
vitamin B-1. See Thiamine
vitamin B-2, 142, 152
vitamin B-6, 150–51, 156
vitamin B-12, 143, 148–50, 156, 208
  by injection, 176
vitamin C, 148, 153, 155, 156
vitamin D, 156
vitamin E, 153–55, 208
vitamins, 148–56
Vivaldi, 78
voltaren, 168
vomeropherins, 33

walking, 52, 69, 71–72
Walking Straight Line test, 52

Warm, Joel, 117
washing car, 69
washing machines, 30
water and salt balance, 33
Waynbaum, Israel, 199
weather stripping, 30
Weizmann Institute, 37, 120, 211
Wernicke's area, 7, 119
Wernicke's encephalopathy, 152
Whipple, Beverly, 81–82
Who Gets Sick? (Pennebaker), 123–24
"Why Stress Is Bad for Your Brain" (Sapolsky), 180
widowers, 184
Wiesel, Torsten, 18
Williams, Mark, 53
Wilson, Edgar, 187
Wilson, Frank, 74–75, 88
Wilson, Matthew, 120
windows, 25, 30
winning, 201
women, and PET scans, 2
woodwinds, 87
work efficiency, 65
"working memory," 93
World Health Organization, 10
writer's block, 134
writing
  Letter to Yourself from Someone Else exercise, 130
  movements and, 47
  and stress, 124

Yenawine, Philip, 113
yoga, 191, 199
Yogman, Michael, 141
"Y" Words exercise, 129

Zatorre, Robert, 77–78
zinc, 157
Zjonc, R. B., 19

0-595-30092-8

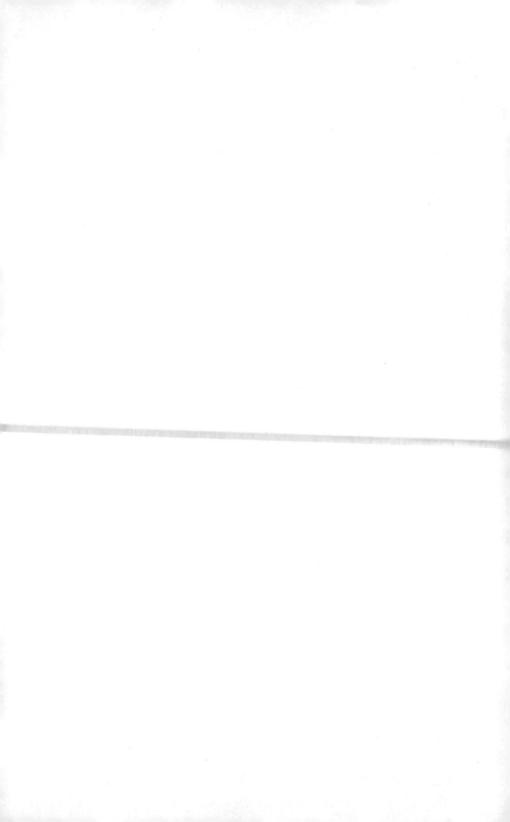